The Hepatitis E Mastery Bible: Your Blueprint for Complete Hepatitis E Management

Dr. Ankita Kashyap and Prof. Krishna N. Sharma

Published by Virtued Press, 2023.

THE HEPATITIS E MASTERY BIBLE: YOUR BLUEPRINT FOR COMPLETE HEPATITIS E MANAGEMENT

First edition. November 20, 2023.

Copyright © 2023 Dr. Ankita Kashyap and Prof. Krishna N. Sharma.

ISBN: 979-8223528890

Written by Dr. Ankita Kashyap and Prof. Krishna N. Sharma.

Table of Contents

....1

The Silent Intruder 2

The Unseen Threat 3

Unmasking the Culprit 6

The Invisible Enemy 9

Dancing With Danger 12

Unmasking the Symptoms 15

The Silent Intruder 16

The Flu's Evil Twin 19

The Unseen Threat 21

The Masked Warrior 24

The Battle Within 27

The Call for Help 30

Diagnostic Dilemmas 32

The Elusive Virus 33

Unmasking the Silent Invader 36

The Lab's Puzzle Pieces 39

Navigating the Diagnostic Maze 42

Holistic Health 45

Unveiling the Power of Holistic Healing 46

Nourishing the Temple: The Healing Power of Nutrition 49

Moving Towards Vitality: Exercise for Hepatitis E
Management 52

The Mind-Body Connection: Cultivating Mindfulness 55

Unlocking the Healing Power of Nature: Herbal Remedies 58

Medication Matters 61

The Antiviral Arsenal 62

The Battle of Immunity 66

Navigating Side Effects 69

Beyond Medication: Holistic Approaches 72

The Future of Hepatitis E Treatment 76

Navigating Nutrition 79

The Power of Nutrient-Rich Foods 80

Unmasking the Hidden Culprits 83

The Art of Meal Planning 86

Supercharged Smoothies and Juices 89

The Healing Symphony of Herbs and Spices 91

Mind Over Matter 94

The Hidden Power of the Mind 95

Unraveling the Stress-Disease Connection 97

The Emotion Epidemic 100

The Mindful Path to Healing 102

Unlocking the Mind-Body Connection 105

The Healing Power of Positive Psychology 108

Finding Strength in Community 111

Building a Support Network 114

Finding Your Tribe 115

Support Groups: A Lifeline 118

The Power of Online Communities 121

Nurturing Personal Relationships 124

Self-Care: A Foundation of Support 126

Navigating Stigma and Discrimination 129

Lifestyle Modifications 132

The Battle Against the Bottle 133

The Hidden Dangers of Alcohol 136

Clearing the Smoke 139

Breaking Free From the Smoking Trap 142

Fueling Your Body With Nutrition 145

Unmasking the Impact of Stress 148

Exercise: Your Liver's Best Friend 150

Nutrition: Fueling Your Liver for Success 153

Stress Less, Live More 156

Exercise: Moving Towards Healing 158

The Power of Exercise 161

Unleashing the Healing Power Within 162
A Dance With Endorphins 165
Reviving the Liver With Movement 167
The Immune Booster Workout 170
Finding Joy in Movement 172
The Journey of a Thousand Steps 175
Coping With Challenges 178
The Rollercoaster of Emotions 179
Finding Strength in Vulnerability 181
Navigating the Dark Days 184
Adapting to a New Normal 187
The Power of Support 190
Embracing Moments of Joy 193
Integrative Therapies 196
The Ancient Art of Acupuncture 197
Herbal Remedies: Nature's Healing Power 200
The Mind-Body Connection: Harnessing Your Inner Healing
Power 202
The Role of Nutritional Therapy in Hepatitis E
Management 205
Exploring Traditional Chinese Medicine 208
Empowerment Through Education 211
The Power of Knowledge 212
Navigating the Healthcare Maze 214
Building a Support Network 217
Unleashing Your Inner Advocate 219
Educating Others: Spreading Awareness 222
Overcoming Stigma 224
Unmasking the Hidden Pain 225
Breaking the Shackles of Shame 227
Embracing Vulnerability 230
The Healing Power of Compassion 233
Forging Resilience in the Face of Judgment 236

Thriving With Hepatitis E..238

The Power of Mindset 239

Setting Meaningful Goals...242

Discovering Passions and Pursuing Joy.........................245

Finding Support and Building a Community 247

Embracing Self-Care and Wellness................................250

Navigating Relationships and Communication.............253

Celebrating Victories and Milestones 256

Embracing Uncertainty and Finding Resilience............259

Healing From Within..264

The Healing Journey Begins...265

The Power of Mind-Body Connection 268

Self-Care: Nurturing the Soul 271

The Importance of Self-Compassion 273

Unleashing Inner Strength: Overcoming Obstacles 276

Embracing the Power of Community 278

Nurturing Relationships 281

The Fragile Bonds of Friendship....................................282

Love in the Time of Hepatitis E.....................................285

The Family Tapestry...288

Finding Support in Unlikely Places 290

The Healing Power of Compassion 294

From Surviving to Thriving..296

A Glimpse of Darkness...297

Embracing Resilience..300

The Gift of Gratitude..303

Unleashing the Growth Mindset 306

Rewriting the Narrative..309

Living Life to the Fullest...311

Embracing Resilience..314

Unleashing the Resilient Spirit.......................................315

Building Resilience Brick by Brick..................................317

Coping With Setbacks: Bouncing Back Stronger 320

The Power of Mindset: Shifting Perspectives 323

Finding Light in the Darkness: Cultivating Hope 327

Embracing Imperfections: Resilience in Vulnerability............329

Redefining Success: Resilience Beyond Achievements 331

The Ripple Effect: Inspiring Resilience in Others 334

A Brighter Future 337

A Glimpse of Hope 338

Revolutionary Breakthroughs...341

Unveiling the Hidden...344

The Ripple Effect 346

A Ray of Light...349

The Road Ahead 352

DISCLAIMER

The information provided in this book is intended for general informational purposes only. The content is not meant to substitute professional medical advice, diagnosis, or treatment. Always consult with a qualified healthcare provider before making any changes to your diabetes management plan or healthcare regimen.

While every effort has been made to ensure the accuracy and completeness of the information presented, the author and publisher do not assume any responsibility for errors, omissions, or potential misinterpretations of the content. Individual responses to diabetes management strategies may vary, and what works for one person might not be suitable for another.

The book does not endorse any specific medical treatments, products, or services. Readers are encouraged to seek guidance from their healthcare providers to determine the most appropriate approaches for their unique medical conditions and needs.

Any external links or resources provided in the book are for convenience and informational purposes only. The author and publisher do not have control over the content or availability of these external sources and do not endorse or guarantee the accuracy of such information.

Readers are advised to exercise caution and use their judgment when applying the information provided in this book to their own situations. The author and publisher disclaim any liability for any direct, indirect, consequential, or other damages arising from the use of this book and its content.

By reading and using this book, readers acknowledge and accept the limitations and inherent risks associated with implementing the strategies, recommendations, and information contained herein. It is always recommended to consult a qualified healthcare professional for personalized medical advice and care.

The Silent Intruder

The Unseen Threat

Anxiety gnawed at my stomach as I waited for the doctor to deliver the results in the antiseptic white room. As soon as the doctor walked in, I couldn't help but notice the weight in his eyes—a dead giveaway that something wasn't quite right. "I'm sorry to notify you that your test results came back positive for Hepatitis E," he said, his eyes empathetic. A wave of panic shot through me, and my heart fell. How on earth is this possible? I had always taken good care of my health, eating a well-balanced diet and maintaining an active lifestyle. My system was completely shocked to receive this diagnosis.

My head was full of questions, and they were getting louder by the second. How did this virus get on me? Was it anything I drank on my most recent trip? Or was it that eatery I went to last week? I felt like I was being swallowed alive by the uncertainty.

Seeing the pain on my face, Dr. Singh sat down next to me and put a consoling hand on my shoulder. His voice firm, he added, "There are several ways that hepatitis E can be caught." "It can be difficult to identify the precise source of the illness, but right now, we need to concentrate on your rehabilitation."

As we discussed the many phases and possible side effects of Hepatitis E, Dr. Singh reassured me that, with the right care and attention, the majority of infected individuals eventually recover completely. He did, however, emphasise how crucial it was to keep an eye on my liver's condition and to visit a doctor if any alarming symptoms appeared.

The weeks that followed were filled with blood tests, doctor's appointments, and a whole lifestyle makeover. I was introduced to a group of professionals by Dr. Singh, each of whom had a distinct area of expertise in wellness and health. They would be my guides together on this unexpected path to recovery.

I met with Dr. Ankita Kashyap, a kind health and wellness coach, for the first time. As soon as I sat in her comfortable office, I felt like a burden had been removed. With genuine concern, Dr. Kashyap took the time to comprehend my worries and anxieties. She underlined that treating Hepatitis E holistically meant not only taking care of the physical symptoms but also taking care of my mental and emotional health.

For me, Dr. Kashyap created a customised lifestyle change plan that included workout regimens, food suggestions, and stress reduction strategies. She espoused the virtues of a diet abundant in fruits, vegetables, lean meats, whole grains, and other foods found in nature. She also advised me to stay away from processed meals and sugary drinks in order to further protect my liver.

However, it went beyond what I ingested. I was also introduced to the effectiveness of counselling and psychology-related practises by Dr. Kashyap. She gave me a toolkit to help me navigate the uncharted waters of a chronic disease, including writing, deep breathing exercises, meditation, and positive affirmations. She continued after that.

With me, Dr. Kashyap discussed complementary and alternative therapy. My daily practise included acupuncture, yoga, and herbal treatments to support my body's natural healing abilities. I felt empowered and in control of my situation while fighting Hepatitis E because to these methods.

I gradually started to see minor gains in my general state of well-being. Dr. Kashyap's nutritional adjustments and stress-reduction methods gave me a fresh lease on life, increasing my vitality and changing my viewpoint. My liver function was regularly monitored, which allowed for early detection of any possible issues and timely intervention and treatment.

I quickly came to understand that hepatitis E was a cunning enemy that could enter a person's system at any time. But fear and anxiety no longer stopped me because I had knowledge, support, and a committed team of professionals at my disposal. Rather, I used my diagnosis as a springboard for a whole makeover, adopting a wholistic perspective on wellbeing and health.

The road to rehabilitation was fraught with difficulties and was by no means easy. However, as I reflect on those trying days, I am appreciative of the strength and tenacity I found within. This transformation may have been sparked by hepatitis E, but it also helped me live a better, more balanced life.

I'll be sharing with you in the upcoming chapters of this book the priceless insights I discovered while trying to control my hepatitis E. We'll go into the specifics of the infection, how it affects the body, and doable ways to adjust and cope. Think of this book as your compass, helping you to navigate the maze that is hepatitis E. With your help, we will enable you to take charge of your health and create a plan for achieving your ideal level of wellbeing.

Unmasking the Culprit

You won't believe what I found out while doing my investigation! The Hepatitis E virus, or HEV, is not a rare illness found only in remote areas with poor sanitation. No,no. This cunning little virus has spread throughout the world, spreading havoc wherever it comes into contact. It's comparable to a tourist who has a one-way ticket and won't return home.

However, let's go back a little and examine the virus's beginnings. Imagine if the Hepatitis E virus was happily coexisting with wild animals in the prehistoric past, when people were still engaged in hunting and gathering activities. But then something terrible happened: people began eating contaminated meat or touching their own bodily fluids too closely. Before you know it, the virus has jumped ship, started its infectious dance, and is spreading to people. And believe me when I say that this virus is a social butterfly that enjoys extending its wings and interacting with cattle in agricultural civilizations.

Let's go back in time to the Industrial Revolution. Urban locations that are densely populated and lack basic sanitation facilities provide the ideal environment for the spread of this terrible virus. The Hepatitis E virus was the life of the party, resembling a massive, contagious gathering. Poor people who lived in such conditions were sitting ducks for this unseen enemy since sanitation was a foreign notion to them.

Hold on to your hats because globalisation is about to take this virus global. Increased trade and travel have made the Hepatitis E virus a frequent traveller. It says "Bon journey!" aboard aeroplanes before causing mayhem in new places. It's spreading throughout nations like wildfire, resembling a virus on steroids. Like a gripping tale that is just waiting to be discovered, every location has a distinct storey to tell about infection rates and transmission.

But be careful—this virus is a cunning little demon. It takes some time to reveal its true colours. It frequently results in a painful episode of acute hepatitis, but it can also cause chronic infection by hanging out in your body. And you know who's most at risk from this enduring bug? those whose immune systems are compromised. Just put that on the list of difficulties we have in eradicating this virus—as if we needed one more twist!

Not to mention that this virus is very expert at disguising itself. It has eight faces instead of only one! You read correctly: there are eight different genotypes, each with a different genetic make-up and degree of nastiness. It seems as though the virus attended a costume party and returned wearing different disguises. Finding a vaccine or treatment becomes a wild goose chase with all these various looks.

What are the secrets to breaking the code of this virus, then? It is out that inadequate hygiene, tainted water supplies, and poor sanitation are important contributors to its spread. It seems the ideal recipe for catastrophe, ready to be mixed and served. As if that weren't enough, raw or undercooked meat from diseased animals—such as deer and wild boars—also acts as an unappealing means of spread. Yikes!

How therefore do we defeat this intruder who is silent? It will require a plethora of ways. First and foremost, we must improve the infrastructure for sanitary conditions, raise public awareness of proper food handling procedures, and educate people about this virus and its transmission. Not to mention immunisation campaigns for susceptible populations, such as expectant mothers and people with compromised immune systems.

It has been a wild ride to delve deeply into the intricacies of this illness, but I'm so pleased I did! Based on my investigation and several discussions with specialists, I have discovered the beginnings and development of the Hepatitis E virus. Equipped with this acquired understanding, I can now devise tactics to oversee and treat my patients with authority.

Don't worry, my dear reader—we're not quite done yet. I'll get into the specifics of diagnosing hepatitis E in the upcoming chapter. I will be divulging all the juicy data regarding the tests and methods that can assist us in detecting this cunning virus and stopping it in its tracks. You'll be on the edge of your seat with a dash of suspense thanks to case studies and personal narratives. So grab a seat, and let's conquer and master Hepatitis E management together!

The Invisible Enemy

You have to see what I found out while doing my study! HEV, commonly known as the hepatitis E virus, is not a rare illness found only in remote areas with poor hygiene. No,no. With its cunning small size, this virus has spread around the world, inflicting havoc wherever it touches. It is comparable to a tourist with a one-way ticket who declines to return home.

Let us examine the history of this virus and go back a little. Imagine if the Hepatitis E virus was happy and unaffected in wild animals back in the prehistoric era, when humans were still engaged in hunting and gathering. Then, however, catastrophe struck: people began consuming contaminated meat or becoming overly intimate with one another's bodily fluids. The virus then proceeds to breach its vessel and initiates its infectious dance, infecting humans in the process. And this virus is a social butterfly, I assure you; it enjoys interacting with cattle in agricultural cultures and extending its reach.

Advance to the era of the Industrial Revolution. This deadly virus found the ideal breeding habitat in densely populated metropolitan areas where basic hygiene standards were lacking. The Hepatitis E virus was enjoying the time of its life at what seemed like a huge, contagious party. The idea of sanitation was alien to them, and the unfortunate people who had to live in such conditions were easy targets for this unseen enemy.

Get ready to embrace globalisation as it embarks on a global tour spreading this illness. The Hepatitis E virus has spread widely due to increased trade and travel. It jumps on aeroplanes and exclaims, "Bon voyage!" before causing mayhem in new places. It's spreading like wildfire, affecting nations all over the world. Every location has a distinct storey to tell about infection rates and transmission, much like a gripping mystery that has yet to be solved.

However, beware—this virus is a cunning little devil. It takes a while to reveal its actual colours. Though it frequently results in a painful episode of acute hepatitis, it can also remain in your body and cause chronic infection. You know who's especially susceptible to this enduring virus, too? Individuals having compromised immune systems. Just add that to the list of difficulties in eradicating this virus—as if we needed one more unexpected turn of events!

Oh, and don't forget that this malware is an expert impersonator. It is not a single face; it has eight! Eight different genotypes, each with a specific genetic make-up and degree of nastiness—yes, you read that right. It's as if the virus attended a masquerade party and returned wearing different personas. It becomes a wild goose hunt to locate a vaccine or treatment with all these diverse looks.

What are the mysteries of this virus that need to be unlocked? As it happens, inadequate hygiene, tainted water sources, and poor sanitation all contribute significantly to its spread. It's like the ideal formula for catastrophe, ready to be unleashed. If that wasn't enough, one pretty unappealing method of transmission is through raw or undercooked meat from infected animals, such as deer and wild boars. Yikes!

How therefore do we defeat this quiet invader? An army of approaches will be required. Building better hygienic infrastructure, promoting safe food handling procedures, and educating the public about this virus and its transmission mechanisms should be our first priorities. Furthermore, vaccination campaigns for susceptible populations—such as expectant mothers and people with compromised immune systems—must not be overlooked.

It's been quite the journey to delve deeply into the secrets of this virus, but I'm so pleased I did! I've learned about the beginnings and development of the Hepatitis E virus through my research and several discussions with specialists. With my improved understanding, I can now devise plans to effectively manage and take care of my patients.

Do not worry, my dear reader; our adventure is far from ended. I'll go into great detail about how to diagnose Hepatitis E in the upcoming chapter. I'll be giving away all the juicy details regarding the procedures and tests that can be used to find this cunning virus and stop it in its tracks. To keep you on the edge of your seat, case studies and personal narratives will add a dash of suspense. So grab a seat, and let's conquer and become experts in managing Hepatitis E!

Dancing With Danger

What I discovered while doing my study will astound you! HEV (hepatitis E virus) is not a rare disease found in remote areas with poor sanitation. No,no. Due to its cunning nature, this small virus has spread around the world, creating havoc wherever it goes. The situation might be compared to a tourist who has a one-way ticket and won't return home.

Let's take a moment to go back in time and investigate the virus's beginnings. Imagine this: the hepatitis E virus was happily coexisting with wild animals in the prehistoric past, when people were still engaged in hunting and gathering activities. Unfortunately, things took a turn for the worst when people began eating contaminated meat and touching their own bodily fluids too closely. The virus suddenly leaves the ship, starts its infectious dance, and infects everyone. And this virus, believe me, is a social butterfly that enjoys extending its wings and interacting with livestock in agricultural communities.

The Industrial Revolution is now in the past. This terrible virus found the ideal environment to grow because of crowded urban areas and a lack of basic hygiene methods. Hepatitis E virus was having a blast at what seemed like a massive, contagious party. People living in such conditions were easy targets for this unseen enemy since sanitation was an alien idea to them.

Tie your laces together, for globalisation is about to take this virus global. The Hepatitis E virus is now widely dispersed due to increased trade and travel. Before inflicting devastation in new locations, it boards flights and exclaims, "Bon voyage!" Reminiscent of a viral pandemic, it is ravaging nations worldwide. Like an intriguing novel waiting to be revealed, every location has an own storey of infection rates and transmission.

A warning, though: this virus is a cunning little devil. True colours don't emerge immediately. It can cause chronic infection in your body, even though it frequently results in a painful episode of acute hepatitis. Who is more susceptible to this enduring bug, by the way? immune system-compromised individuals. Like we needed another curveball! Just add that to the list of difficulties in battling this infection!

Furthermore, this virus is very expert at disguising itself. There are eight faces on it instead of just one! Yeah, you read correctly: there are eight different genotypes, each with a different genetic make-up and degree of ugliness. It seems like the virus assumed several personas and returned from a costume party. Searching for a vaccination or treatment becomes a fruitless endeavour with so many variations in appearance.

Thus, what are the secrets of being able to unlock this virus? The prevalence of it is largely attributed to inadequate hygiene, tainted water sources, and poor sanitation. It's as if the ideal formula for catastrophe is there, ready to explode. Even more unappealing is the fact that raw or undercooked meat from sick animals, such as deer and wild boars, can spread the infection. Yikes!

What then is the best way to eliminate this quiet invader? An army of approaches will be necessary. Improved food handling procedures must be promoted, improved sanitation infrastructure must be built, and the general public must be educated about this virus and its transmission. Additionally, we must remember to vaccinate susceptible populations, such as individuals with compromised immune systems and pregnant women.

Though it has been a wild ride, I'm so glad I took the time to delve deeply into the intricacies of this virus! I now know the history and evolution of the hepatitis E virus thanks to my research and several discussions with specialists. I can now handle and take care of my patients like a boss because of the knowledge I have gained.

Moreover, our voyage is far from over, so relax, dear reader. The specifics of diagnosing Hepatitis E will be covered in detail in the upcoming chapter. All the juicy details regarding the tests and methods that can help us find this cunning virus and stop it in its tracks will be revealed by me. A dash of suspense to keep you on the edge of your seat will come from case studies and personal tales. As we conquer and perfect the management of Hepatitis E, please buckle up and join me!

Unmasking the Symptoms

The Silent Intruder

Allow me to share with you this amazing tale that has stayed with me. It concerns Maya, this young lady. Envision her, in her mid-twenties, exuberant and carefree. She had no idea that a straightforward Hepatitis E diagnosis would have such a profound impact.

Maya didn't give it much thought at first. Hey, it's just a slight illness, no big issue, she thought to herself. She had no idea, though, that her carefree demeanour would come back to bite her in the worst way.

Maya began to feel more and more exhausted with time. She was often tired, had lost her appetite, and even became jaundiced. But what did she do, you know? She dismissed it, assuming it was just one of life's normal ups and downs. How incorrect, oh, she was.

Things became much worse for her. Maya started to have severe abdominal pain, her body bloated with fluid, and tests on her liver function revealed some significant damage. If she had taken her Hepatitis E seriously, she could have prevented the progression of the illness to chronic liver disease.

Could you envision? This virus infiltrated her liver, resulting in scarring and inflammation that would harm this vital organ irreversibly. When Maya's condition deteriorated, a liver transplant was her only chance of survival. The ramifications of her casual attitude are devastating.

Maya is not alone, though. I'd like to introduce you to Rajesh, a man in his middle age whose storey is equally heartbreaking. Rajesh was a dedicated family man who was always balancing a lot of obligations. He didn't hesitate to put his health on the back burner after learning he had Hepatitis E during a routine checkup.

Years passed, and Rajesh ignored the ticking time bomb inside of him as he continued living his life. And then one day he passed out at work. He was suddenly afflicted with acute liver failure. While they battled valiantly to save him, the doctors' chances of survival were slim. A liver transplant was his sole remaining chance.

Thank goodness, Maya and Rajesh were both fortunate enough to have the much-needed transplants. However, their tales serve as a sobering reminder of the perils associated with hepatitis E neglect. They could have saved themselves from all of this pain if they had only asked for assistance sooner. It serves as a reminder to all of us of the value of routine examinations, self-education regarding the illness, and never holding off on seeking medical assistance when something is wrong.

You see, if Hepatitis E is not treated, it can result in a variety of consequences. It may result in liver failure, a potentially fatal condition. Furthermore, if it persists for a long time, your liver may become severely scarred and unable to function. Imagine the accumulation of fluid, the internal bleeding, and the elevated risk of liver cancer. It scares me.

It is imperative that we recognise the seriousness of Hepatitis E. It acts as if it were a cunning intruder, silently destroying our liver without our knowledge. It may already be too late by the time we become aware of the symptoms.

So, how can we guard against this Hepatitis E tightrope walk? It all comes down to being proactive, though. Vaccinate yourself if you reside in a region where this virus is prevalent. Pay attention to hygiene, particularly in relation to food and water. Additionally, remember to fully cook your meat. Frequent examinations and screenings can identify the virus early on, allowing us to combat it head-on.

These first-hand accounts vividly illustrate the possible repercussions of disregarding Hepatitis E. They serve as a constant reminder of how crucial it is to identify problems early, take prompt action, and maintain ongoing care in order to stop more complications. We can avoid tripping over this tightrope and allowing Hepatitis E to wreck our lives if we remain knowledgeable, stay on top of things, and take our healthcare seriously.

So keep in mind, dear friend: you are responsible for your own health. Hepatitis E shouldn't cause you to lose your equilibrium. Remain composed, remain knowledgeable, and take charge of your life.

The Flu's Evil Twin

Chapter 4: The Flu's Evil Twin

So, as a medical doctor and health and wellness coach, here I am, sitting down to discuss with you a long-standing concern of mine. Patients who arrive with symptoms that appear to be severe flu-like symptoms only to find that there is something far more terrible going on underneath the surface is something I see far too frequently. You should know that it's like the evil twin of the flu.

The moniker Hepatitis E belongs to this evil twin. Hepatitis A, B, and C are some of their more well-known siblings, but this cunning one frequently remains untreated. It is a virus that occasionally masquerades as the flu or a normal cold. Health care providers are unable to distinguish it because of how effectively it blends in.

The fact is that there can be some similarities between the symptoms of the flu and Hepatitis E. You have flu-like symptoms, including fever, lethargy, and aches in your muscles. This is where things can get complicated, though, because hepatitis E prefers to act like a transient virus that will go away on its own. And that's when it begins to silently and unnoticeably wreck havoc on your liver.

Imagine having a little temperature, a sore throat, and a runny nose as you wake up. It seems like a regular cold, so you dismiss it and get on with your day. But these sensations merely keep getting worse as the days stretch into weeks. You begin to feel quite exhausted as they get stronger. Next appear the characteristic symptoms of a serious liver problem: jaundice, black urine, and pale faeces.

There's a sense of urgency for a diagnosis since by this time the damage might already be done. That being said, here's the issue: it's nearly impossible to distinguish between hepatitis E and the flu. You may easily write off hepatitis E as another flu episode because they are so similar. That's why it's critical that those of us working in the healthcare industry are alert, ask probing questions, and do the required testing. It is imperative that we apprehend this malevolent twin before it causes permanent harm.

Persistence is one feature that distinguishes Hepatitis E from the flu. The duration of Hepatitis E might persist for weeks or even months, in contrast to the week or so that the flu can linger. That is a telltale symptom of a problem. When your flu-like symptoms become more persistent, perhaps even bothersome, it's time to think about Hepatitis E and see a doctor.

As I have personally witnessed, postponing diagnosis and treatment can have disastrous consequences. I feel so sorry for the patients, their livers, and themselves. all due to the evil twin's prolonged absence from sight. My guys, we must lift our game. To ensure that nobody becomes a victim of this cunning adversary, we must increase awareness and educate ourselves.

I would like you to understand that Hepatitis E is a serious illness, to sum up. Though it's much more than the flu, it deceives us into believing that it is. Our vigilance must be maintained, particularly during those prolonged episodes of flu-like symptoms. Acknowledging its true nature and responding promptly with diagnosis and treatment can help us combat this evil sibling. We can fend off the flu's cunning and dangerous twin by banding together to safeguard ourselves and our loved ones.

The Unseen Threat

You know, the first thing that typically comes to mind when thinking about Hepatitis E is polluted water. Water is, after all, practically necessary for our survival, right? It is the source of our continued existence. However, what occurs if that safety net is compromised? When this unseen attacker uses it as a breeding ground? Unbelievably, tainted water is a major source of Hepatitis E infection in many regions of the world, particularly in countries with inadequate sanitation facilities. For example, it occurs when sewage seeps into sources of drinking water or when individuals disregard basic hygiene, such as not cleaning their hands after using the restroom. Could you picture that? This terrible virus can infect you for something as trivial as not washing your hands.

The really bad news is this. Not just water poses a risk. This invisible threat can even be present in the food we eat. Were you aware that undercooked or uncooked meat can spread Hepatitis E? Yes, especially wild game and pork. Even though the animals appear healthy, the virus can persist in infected animals and their organs. Thus, disaster strikes if you handle or cook tainted meat improperly! You can be giving yourself or your loved ones the Hepatitis E virus. This is the reason I, as a health and wellness coach, constantly emphasise to my patients the significance of safe eating habits. such as utilising appropriate cooking methods and steering clear of undercooked or raw meats. Folks, this is not a joke.

We've talked about food and water, now let's talk about this. The air we breathe has the potential to spread hepatitis E. Yes, I realise that it sounds like something from a horror film. It turns out that the virus can remain on surfaces for an absurdly long period of time, and that it can spread via the air when those surfaces are disturbed. Thus, seemingly innocuous objects like doorknobs or shared cutlery might harbour that virulent virus and spread it to unwary individuals. And believe me when I say that the risk of airborne transmission skyrockets in locations with inadequate ventilation, such as crowded public transit or small areas. Very eerie stuff, huh? especially considering that hepatitis E can silently spread among a large population without any symptoms.

While knowing how this virus spreads is useful, what really counts is taking precautions to keep ourselves and our loved ones safe. Even though hepatitis E is invisible, we still have options for resistance. Having access to safe and clean drinking water is one of the best strategies to prevent infection. We require the implementation of appropriate water treatment and sanitation systems. And let's not overlook the significance of teaching everyone how to properly wash their hands. People, that's a big one.

We also need to exercise caution when it comes to diet. To do this, use safe food handling and cooking methods. You know, cleaning and sanitising our produce, fully cooking meat to eliminate any possible bacteria, and, for the love of all that is good, refraining from eating raw or undercooked meat. particularly if we have doubts about the source. Yes, it might sound painful, but at least it's not as bad as contracting hepatitis E, right?

And let's not overlook the importance of personal hygiene. That also matters a lot. It's imperative to regularly wash your hands with soap and water, especially after using the restroom or handling potentially contaminated objects. Those germs are gone, people. Furthermore, let's remember to clean and sanitise everything like sharing utensils and doorknobs. Even though we might not give them much thought, they might be carrying that unseen threat.

I constantly remind my patients that prevention is the key as a health and wellness consultant, you know? It goes beyond simply cleaning and avoiding things. It's about looking after ourselves as a whole. Hence, maintaining a healthy lifestyle, engaging in regular exercise, eating a balanced diet, and getting adequate sleep can all help to boost our immune systems and reduce our susceptibility to illnesses. Indeed, stress management and self-care practises are equally crucial. My friends, it's all about enhancing our general resilience and well-being.

Let's conclude now. Hepatitis E resembles this cunning little adversary that lurks in unexpected places. It is present in the foods we eat, the water we drink, and even the air we breathe. Strange, huh? But fear not—we are capable of retaliation. We may defeat this unseen foe by having access to clean water, handling food safely, practising good personal hygiene, and approaching our health holistically. All we need to do is bring it to light and equip ourselves with information and safeguards. Now is the time to take Hepatitis E to task!

The Masked Warrior

You know, you have to know what this infection is all about if you really want to understand the hardships that individuals with Hepatitis E face. Therefore, Hepatitis E is essentially a viral infection of the liver (HEV). These days, it's a cunning little pest that likes to spread through tainted food or water. That's the reason it's so important in areas with poor hygiene and sanitation standards. Not only that, but this sucker may also be passed from mother to unborn child and through blood transfusions. Admit it—you are obstinate.

In contrast to other forms of viral hepatitis, hepatitis E typically resolves on its own. That basically indicates that most people can recover on their own in a matter of weeks or months. However, I must warn you that for many unfortunate individuals, the road to recovery can truly resemble a rollercoaster.

Let's take a closer look at the thirty-five-year-old mother of two, Katherine. Katherine, poor Katherine, contracted hepatitis E while expecting her second child. She didn't even exhibit any symptoms at first, and her blood testing appeared normal. However, she suddenly began to feel as though a truck had ran her over. You name it: nausea and fatigue. At that point, she recognised she needed assistance.

Katherine can still clearly recall those initial days following her diagnosis. Says she, "I felt like I was taken out by surprise. It didn't even occur to me that I had Hepatitis E until I was informed that I did. I was so afraid for my child, afraid of what it would do to him. The doctor tried to reassure me, telling me there was little risk of injury. However, you know, that dread is difficult to overcome."

As time passed, Katherine discovered that she was suffering from the mental and physical effects of having Hepatitis E. She was unable to care for her newborn or fulfil her other obligations due to the exhaustion, which was overwhelming her like a tidal wave. "Even something as easy as cooking dinner or giving my infant a bath felt like scaling Mount Everest. I had to constantly tell myself that I was fighting a damn war even though it seemed like I was failing as a mother. I had to put all of my energy into fighting my way back and have faith in my family."

Though Katherine's experience exemplifies tremendous willpower, let me assure you that she's not alone. This exploration of the world of Hepatitis E introduces us to Mark, a young, ambitious man who contracted the illness while travelling overseas. The poor guy found it quite difficult to receive a diagnosis. He was suffering from extreme tiredness, anorexia, and very dark urine. But what did they say, you know? Aircraft lag. I mean, really? Mark didn't receive medical attention until his condition deteriorated and the jaundice set in.

Mark muses over those difficult times and says, "That never-ending dance of weakness and exhaustion was what really caught me off guard. There were moments when I thought I would never be able to get out of bed. This really got to me because I've always considered myself to be a driven someone with a lot of life. To even get close to normal again, it required months of adjusting my lifestyle and learning self-care."

We begin to understand the extraordinary bravery that arises when life hands you a raw deal through the experiences of Katherine and Mark. They had to contend with mental conflicts that caused them to doubt everything as well as physical challenges that drove them to the verge. However, they unearthed a strength they never thought they had during that fight.

But here's the deal. Not everyone has hepatitis E in the same way. Some people heal quickly and only have minor symptoms. Some are not as fortunate. Their recovery will take longer and be more difficult. For this reason, treating Hepatitis E holistically is essential. It is imperative that we attend to these soldiers' emotions and mental health in addition to their bodily needs.

We'll delve further into each facet of managing hepatitis E in the upcoming chapters. We will cover topics such as dietary modifications, psychology and therapy, self-help techniques, and coping mechanisms. We can defend ourselves and take action when our own health is in jeopardy by learning from people who have confronted this unseen foe.

Hepatitis E may appear to be a minor illness, but underneath that mask, as you will see, it exposes the bravery and tenacity of people who face it head-on. Through their experiences, we are able to access the inner strength that everyone of us possesses to overcome any obstacle and become independent warriors.

The Battle Within

Hi everyone! I have dedicated my professional life to exploring the realm of holistic healthcare and wellness as a medical doctor and health and wellness coach. Furthermore, Hepatitis E is not to be taken lightly. Given the devastating effects this virus can have on our bodies, it's critical to comprehend the fierce internal struggle that results from infection. I promise that we can defeat Hepatitis E like champions if we know how our body responds to infection and how to control our immune system.

Let's now discuss the immune system. Imagine it as this intricate team of tissues, cells, and organs defending our bodies from dangerous intruders. Our immune system kicks in when a cunning Hepatitis E virus decides to spoil the fun. It's prepared to kick some viral butt, akin to a fast response squad. Our mighty macrophages eat away at the Hepatitis E virus in an effort to destroy it before it has a chance to propagate and wreak havoc. These heroes take quick action to minimise the damage and limit the infection.

That's not all, though. These signalling molecules, also known as cytokines, are released by our innate immune system. Consider them as messengers alerting the army to the impending invasion of viruses. Other immune cells can launch a more focused onslaught with this heads-up. In the fight against Hepatitis E, the immune system is leading the way, much like in a choreographed dance.

The adaptive immune system is now present. This mechanism functions similarly to the brains underlying both targeted viral elimination and long-term immunity. Our adaptive immune system summons the big guns—T cells—when Hepatitis E chooses to persist. These men are the immune army's foot soldiers. Before the virus has a chance to spread, they are able to detect and eliminate the contaminated cells. Hepatitis E and T cells are engaged in a bloody struggle where both are always changing their tactics.

And you know what? We have additional support at our disposal. When B cells arrive, they start to produce these potent proteins known as antibodies. They recognise and attach only to the Hepatitis E virus, much like intelligent missiles. These antibodies not only neutralise the virus but also identify it so that other immune cells can destroy it. Talk about cooperation, huh?

The adaptive immune response resembles this amazing coalition of several cell types cooperating flawlessly to eradicate the pathogen. The ways in which our immune system changes and adapts to defeat Hepatitis E is astounding. Hold on, though—the battle hasn't ended yet. This virus is cunning; it may adapt to outwit our immune system by hiding inside cells or by changing. However, our immune system is resilient and doesn't give up easy. It keeps fighting and invents new strategies to stay one step ahead.

There's something more to this internal struggle we have. Our immune system is a formidable force that demonstrates remarkable flexibility and resilience. It resembles a complex web of defence mechanisms, signalling chemicals, and cells working together to thwart the Hepatitis E virus.

It's exciting and powerful to know how our immune system reacts to hepatitis E. Equipped with this understanding, we may actively aid our immune system in combating the infection. You know, basic habits like eating healthily, getting enough sleep, controlling stress, and maintaining an active lifestyle can all support a stronger immune system. Additionally, supplementary and alternative therapies like herbal medicines, acupuncture, and meditation may provide you a competitive advantage.

So let's embark together on this adventure to learn all there is to know about controlling Hepatitis E and to identify the most effective methods and instruments for curing this illness. By working together, we may discover the solutions for managing Hepatitis E completely and create the foundation for a happier, healthier future. Hurry up, let's get started!

The Call for Help

Folks, I've personally witnessed it. Hepatitis E is not your typical viral illness that plays havoc with your body. No, it's a severe illness that permeates every part of your existence. You experience a plethora of horrible symptoms, such as excruciating stomach ache, eyes and skin yellowing, and bone-crushing exhaustion. However, that's not even the worst part—the really mind-bender is what transpires within your skull.

Feeling the symptoms of Hepatitis E is like being on a roller coaster in your brain, with anxiety and bewilderment riding shotgun. You're left dashing around, attempting to make sense of all the strange physical changes that have occurred. That is the moment when your soul begins to ring with alarms, calling for help to arrive.

Seeking assistance can resemble attempting to scale Mount Everest. You hesitate because of the ridiculous stigma associated with contagious diseases—you don't want people to know what you're going through. You eventually start to feel like a lone ship lost at sea as feelings of shame and embarrassment seep in.

Friends, here's the thing: asking for medical assistance is never a show of weakness. It takes courage to seek for the assistance you need and face the music. Early detection and management of Hepatitis E is essential for managing its horrible symptoms and preventing complications. So, I promise you, see a medical professional about your butt. To set you on the correct route, they are equipped with the appropriate instruments and strategies.

I won't lie to you, though: navigating our healthcare system can be quite the maze. Doctors, appointments, drugs—you can feel your mind spinning. However, don't let it deceive you. Raise your voice and make your needs known. Make sure you receive the high-quality medical treatment you are entitled to and that your voice is heard.

It also makes a huge difference to have a support team. Rely on your friends, family, and loved ones during difficult times. When you most need them, they'll be there to listen, wipe away your tears, and offer support. Through thick and thin, you can rely on them.

Additionally, remember about you. Yes, you do matter. Friend, treat yourself with kindness. It's a long and uneven path to rehabilitation, but you must remain positive. Be kind to yourself; eat healthily, get exercise, engage in activities that uplift your spirits. And counselling? Before you judge it, give it a try. You'd be shocked at how much of an impact it may have on your emotional health.

Let me tell you as a health and wellness coach: taking a comprehensive approach is crucial. Yes, it is crucial to cure the physical symptoms, but the work doesn't end there. The psychological and emotional issues also need to be addressed. That entails providing you with all the equipment and tactics need to take on this beast. It's about assuming responsibility and ruling your own happiness and health.

There you have it, then. Hepatitis E is more than just a sickness; it's a cry for assistance that goes unanswered. It begs for sympathy, understanding, and assistance. We may force Hepatitis E to comply with our wishes by recognising the emotional aspect of the disease and providing you with all the resources you require to cope with it. Together, we'll make sense of the complex healthcare system and design a plan to permanently eradicate Hepatitis E.

Diagnostic Dilemmas

The Elusive Virus

I will never forget the day Mrs. Wilson entered my clinic, her body burdened by a multitude of ailments and her face etched with tiredness. She reported having constant nausea, exhaustion, and appetite loss. You know, the kind that makes you feel like a deflated balloon on a beautiful morning that gnaws at your stomach. As a physician who is passionate about providing holistic care, I was aware that a wide range of medical conditions may be the source of these symptoms.

But then, like a flash in the darkness, something drew my attention. Mrs. Wilson's liver enzymes were alarmingly singing for attention when I did some standard tests. I couldn't help but think of "Hepatitis E," a virus that is known to severely damage the liver. However, the challenge proved trickier to solve than I had thought. The prankster hepatitis E likes to lurk in plain sight, frequently masquerading as other illnesses due to its characteristics. It makes sense why they refer to it as the "silent epidemic."

It was evident to me as I dug into Mrs. Wilson's medical history and began to piece things together like a detective on a case that her path had been a convoluted web of incorrect diagnoses and unsuccessful therapies. She was physically and emotionally exhausted, as other medical professionals had overlooked the Hepatitis E marker. Seeing the toll it had taken on her, both physically and mentally, crushed my heart.

However, I wasn't prepared to give up just yet. Oh no, Mr. Armed with vials of blood, mountains of tests, and a voracious appetite for answers, I set out on a ceaseless quest for the truth. We examined and examined, probing and poking, in the hopes that every test would cast a light on the shadows. However, the outcomes frequently played ambiguous, leaving us perplexed and increasing Mrs. Wilson's irritation.

Further complicating our search were the potential co-infections or underlying diseases that we could not rule out. It resembled fighting a shape-shifting monster since every turn revealed a new aspect and obstacle to conquer.

However, the realm of inquiry and scholarly books provided comfort for my thoughts despite my frustration. I read a tonne of medical papers, digested conference insights, and talked to other authorities in the field for advice. The more I learned about the complexity of Hepatitis E, the more I understood that it was a complex web of mystery and intrigue as much as a medical issue.

Every Hepatitis E patient seems to have a different narrative to tell, a different set of symptoms and circumstances. It resembled attempting to solve a puzzle with an infinite number of possible solutions. The virus was an expert at trickery; it could pass for other liver disorders or sneak past people's attention.

Furthermore, upon stepping foot in the realm of healthcare professionals, I learned that Mrs. Wilson's ordeal was not an exceptional one. Similar challenges had been encountered by other people before receiving a Hepatitis E diagnosis. It was obvious that understanding this virus's evasive character was essential to raising diagnostic precision and, eventually, patient outcomes.

But even in the midst of this difficult journey, I saw something amazing: the tenacity and unyielding spirit of patients such as Mrs. Wilson. They clung to optimism like a lifeline in spite of the disappointments and defeats. They gave me the motivation to keep going, to keep looking for solutions, and to stand up for them in this difficult fight.

As my knowledge increased, I came to understand that treating Hepatitis E involved more than just combating the infection directly. No, it was not only that. It required a comprehensive strategy and an awareness of how important it was to determine vulnerability to infection from the underlying causes. Dietary planning, lifestyle adjustments, and psychiatric counselling all became crucial components of the jigsaw. To help our patients on their journey to wellbeing, I assembled a team that included dietitians, psychologists, and practitioners of alternative medicine.

It took what felt like a lifetime, but Mrs. Wilson and I eventually uncovered the truth: Hepatitis E. We were relieved and triumphant in our discovery, but we were also frustrated by the long and convoluted journey that had brought us to this point. Despite everything, though, my determination to enhance the identification and treatment of hepatitis E remained unwavering.

Allow readers of this subchapter to get a glimpse of the elusiveness of hepatitis E. Make them understand that it takes a warrior's spirit to diagnose or simply brush off a virus. Through my personal journey, I hope to highlight the difficulties that both patients and healthcare professionals confront and the value of tenacity and teamwork in solving the riddles of this silent pandemic.

Unmasking the Silent Invader

Imagine one morning waking up completely exhausted, as though everything had been taken from you. It's a fatigue that follows you around, regardless of how much sleep you've had. You persevere through the day, assuming your lack of appetite is only a fleeting peculiarity and that perhaps it's just a passing lethargy. However, during the course of the following few days, the tiredness worsens and is accompanied by a moderate temperature, achy joints, and sporadic nausea. You begin reaching for over-the-counter drugs in the vain hope that they may provide you with some respite. You have no idea, though, that these seemingly harmless symptoms could be the quiet whispers of a malevolent invader quietly moving in with you.

The liver is the main organ affected by the virus that causes hepatitis E. It spreads by contaminated food or water, particularly in places with inadequate hygiene and sanitation standards. The virus can also be spread by close contact with an infected individual. But what really makes Hepatitis E so sneaky is its capacity to hide, going long stretches without being seen.

As a physician and a health and fitness coach, I have personally seen how nimble Hepatitis E can be. Its symptoms are so mild that they are easily disregarded or confused with those of other illnesses. This secretive intruder can stealthily progress from the acute to the chronic stage, making diagnosis and treatment even more difficult. However, my goal is to arm you with the knowledge required for early detection and intervention by illuminating these covert indicators.

One of the most prevalent and early signs of Hepatitis E is fatigue. Many people find themselves perpetually exhausted and unable to carry out even the most basic daily duties. They dismiss it, attributing it to stress or a hectic schedule. In addition, once exhaustion sets in, appetite declines, which might lead to inadvertent weight loss. These insignificant-seeming symptoms are frequently written off as normal life's ups and downs, which makes individuals put off getting help until it's too late.

Occasionally, patients and healthcare providers may encounter perplexing challenges due to flu-like symptoms. People frequently turn to self-medication when they have moderate body pains, fever, nausea, and joint pain because they believe it's just the typical flu or a transitory viral infection. They are unaware, however, that Hepatitis E can also mirror identical symptoms, therefore it's important to spot the pattern and seek out more medical testing.

Hepatitis E can have a severe negative impact on mental and emotional health in addition to its physical manifestations. Many people report experiencing mood swings, irritation, and general discomfort. Many times, people ignore these psychological symptoms or mistake them for the effects of outside pressures, which causes delays or incorrect diagnosis. My goal in exposing this silent invader is to draw attention to the connection between mental and physical health and the importance of a comprehensive approach to treatment.

It takes diligence and initiative to spot these subtle indicators in order to expose this stealthy invader. I urge you to be aware of your body, to pay attention to its cues, and to get medical help if something seems even slightly out of the ordinary. Treatment outcomes can be greatly improved and additional complications can be avoided with early identification.

Furthermore, I beg you to put your general wellbeing first. Reduce your chance of contracting Hepatitis E by leading a lifestyle that supports the health of your liver and immune system. Maintaining a healthy diet, exercising frequently, and practising good cleanliness are all essential defences against this cunning intruder. You may improve your body's resistance to infections and fortify your defences by implementing minor changes to your regular routine.

In the pages that follow, I will provide you a step-by-step guide to managing your Hepatitis E. We'll discuss the virus's emotional and psychological effects in addition to its bodily side effects. I think it's important to approach health and wellness from a holistic perspective, encompassing several aspects and enabling you to take charge of your own health.

The lifestyle changes, food and nutrition planning, counselling and psychological approaches, complementary and alternative forms of self-care, and coping mechanisms will all be covered in the upcoming chapters. Adopting this multifaceted strategy will provide you the information and resources you need to manage Hepatitis E successfully.

Together, let's set out on this adventure to uncover the covert symptoms of this silent invader and equip ourselves with the knowledge necessary to see the warning indications and seek prompt medical attention. By working together, we can conquer the management of Hepatitis E and open the door to a happier and healthier future.

The Lab's Puzzle Pieces

I still recall my initial interaction with a patient who was looking for information regarding their diagnosis of hepatitis E. The worry and uncertainty in their eyes reflected the unpredictability of the illness. Being a doctor who treats the patient as a whole, I was aware that deciphering this conundrum would need explaining the laboratory tests.

Let me explain the importance of these tests before we get too technical. They are essential in determining the full scope of the infection and directing the patient's healing process. We enable patients to have an active role in their diagnosis and treatment by integrating them into the process and providing them with understanding of these tests.

Blood tests are the first step in the process, providing a glimpse into the body's internal struggle. These examinations, referred to as liver function tests (LFTs), assess various proteins and enzymes circulating in the blood, offering vital information about the condition of the liver. Increased liver damage or inflammation may be indicated by elevated levels of enzymes such as aspartate aminotransferase (AST) and alanine aminotransferase (ALT), which may indicate the presence of Hepatitis E. Don't overlook the bilirubin levels either. A malfunctioning liver may be the cause of a rise in this tiny troublemaker.

That is, however, merely the tip of the iceberg in the lab. Examining the wider picture necessitates going further into the diagnosis. That's when the exciting part starts.

First, we look for Hepatitis E antibodies, which are little fighters made by the immune system. The blood contains these antibodies, which go by the names immunoglobulin M (IgM) and immunoglobulin G (IgG). As the body fights an acute infection, IgM antibodies are now the first to arrive on the scene. Conversely,

IgG antibodies remain in the body for months or even years following exposure. Healthcare professionals can determine if an infection is current or if the patient has already recovered by assessing the presence and quantity of these antibodies.

Naturally, this diagnostic trip is not as simple as it seems. To uncover the whole tale, sophisticated serologic testing are required.

Let's begin the analysis using reverse transcription polymerase chain reaction (RT-PCR). It may sound absurd, but it's revolutionary. This method allows researchers to identify and multiply the Hepatitis E virus genetic material in a patient's blood. Speaking of investigative work! The infection is brought to light by RT-PCR, even in situations with low viral levels. Because of this, it's especially helpful in exposing long-term Hepatitis E infections that may attempt to evade our army of antibodies.

The test with a rising following is the enzyme-linked immunosorbent assay (ELISA). It works similarly to a magic wand to find particular antibodies that fight Hepatitis E. Serum or stool samples allow ELISA to do its magic and give a more thorough examination of the virus. The best part is that it can even differentiate between various genotypes of Hepatitis E. That small method provides important information on the course and intensity of the infection.

However, that is not where the key to the laboratory kingdom ends. To determine the general health of our Hepatitis E warriors, we still have a few tests up our sleeves.

Red and white blood cell counts are provided by a complete blood count (CBC), which does its magic. This useful tool sheds light on possible physiological effects of the infection. Furthermore, studies using magnetic resonance imaging or ultrasounds to image the liver should not be overlooked (MRI). With the use of these contemporary wonders, we may peer inside the liver to examine its architecture and look for any warning indications of problems.

My colleagues and I never lose sight of the significance of open communication and patient empowerment during this tortuous path. We urge our patients to actively participate in their comprehension of the laboratory tests we perform, to seek clarification, and to ask questions. Patients who comprehend the intent and importance of every test turn into fervent supporters of accurate findings. That's when the true enchantment occurs.

Permit me to illustrate the potential influence that these puzzle pieces can have. I recall a patient who arrived at our office exhibiting the typical signs and symptoms of hepatitis E. The poor creature has been travelling from doctor to doctor and getting its blood tested nonstop. However, the reality wasn't discovered until a thorough panel of serologic testing. Certain antibodies subtly indicated their existence, rendering Hepatitis E unable of remaining concealed. This case demonstrated the value of specialised testing and demonstrated the distinction between striking the target and missing the mark.

Next, a different patient had a false positive for Hepatitis E based only on liver function testing. But we were more aware. We probed further, running more serologic testing, which identified an additional viral infection torturing the liver. We put this patient on the correct track and provided the right therapy and management plan by recognising the limitations of specific diagnostics and doing extensive research.

This laboratory problem is not limited to medical specialists to solve. My intention, dear reader, is to arm you with the information necessary to seek out appropriate diagnoses and ask the proper questions. Equipped with this knowledge, you can actively participate in your healthcare journey and make well-informed choices on your course of treatment. Recall that information is power. One puzzle piece at a time, we'll tackle the complicated world of Hepatitis E diagnosis and treatment together.

Navigating the Diagnostic Maze

I'd like to share a tale with you about a man named Sahil. Imagine a middle-aged man who appears exhausted, grips his stomach, and has hardly opened eyes from lack of sleep. I tell you, it's not a pretty sight. Sahil was currently suffering from the consequences of his recent travel to a location known for having a high rate of Hepatitis E. His body was in a desperate attempt to find relief from the exhaustion, the agony in his abdomen, and most importantly, the yellowing of his skin. Yes, it was just as horrible as it seems.

Sahil took the proper course of action and saw Dr. Patel, his physician. All he could hope for was that Dr. Patel would have the solution to his issues and that at last his symptoms would make sense. And what's this? Dr. Patel quickly concluded that Sahil's problems might be related to Hepatitis E. The results of the liver enzyme test showed increased levels, which may indicate liver damage. However, more testing was required for a definitive diagnosis of Hepatitis E, and that's where things became complicated.

You see, depending on your location and type of healthcare system, the specific tests available for Hepatitis E can vary significantly. In certain regions, the sophisticated testing are limited to reference labs or large hospitals, making correct diagnosis extremely difficult. Fortunately, Dr. Patel was amazing and was able to locate a specialised facility that could perform the tests that Sahil required.

But their problems didn't end there. Oh no, definitely not. It turns out that different laboratories perform Hepatitis E tests and procedures differently, which might produce disparate findings and interpretations. It resembles negotiating an endless maze, where there is increasing uncertainty at every step. Sahil and Dr. Patel needed to be astute and remain at the top of their game.

I could see the frustration written all over Sahil's face during this trip. He was fed up with searching in vain and without solutions. But he persisted in trying. He rolled up his sleeves and became an advocate for himself. He asked a tonne of questions of Dr. Patel, did a tonne of research, and started contributing to every decision that was made. And what's this? Seeing Sahil's commitment, Dr. Patel made a special effort to get him the support he required.

When combined, they posed no threat. They realised the value of working together, utilising all of their resources and bringing in specialists from various fields. They were aware of the shortcomings of the healthcare system, but they also believed that by working together, they could overcome any challenge.

Helen Keller once said, "Alone, we can do so little; together, we can achieve so much." I can't help but think of this. That remark was exemplified by Sahil and Dr. Patel. They realised that arriving at an appropriate diagnosis required collaboration rather than going it alone. They took the problems head-on, admitted that the system was flawed, and battled valiantly to overcome the diagnostic maze.

And what's this? They succeeded. When Sahil received his diagnosis at last, it felt like a triumph against all the odds. It's true that working through the Hepatitis E diagnostic maze is not easy. The scarcity of exams, the differences in approaches, and the mental You may feel like tearing your hair out due to perplexing interpretations. But you can get through that maze and emerge with the proper diagnosis and course of treatment if you never give up, actively engage in your own healthcare decisions, and develop a solid relationship with your healthcare provider.

My eyes were genuinely enlightened to the intricacies of diagnosis by Sahil's experience. It's a tangled network of opportunities rather than a one-way street. It necessitates a multifaceted strategy involving collaboration between medical staff and patients. By sharing my storey, I wish to encourage others to take charge of their health, to keep going when things seem difficult, and to value teamwork in the search for the best possible diagnosis and course of treatment. Although the diagnostic maze may seem overwhelming, we can overcome it as a team.

Holistic Health

Unveiling the Power of Holistic Healing

You know, managing Hepatitis E involves more than just taking medication and calling it a day. There's a lot more to it than just treating the physical symptoms and lowering the virus in your body, which is the emphasis of standard medical therapies. You see, we are more than simply our physical forms—we are also emotional, mental, and spiritual creatures. So, the secret to healing and rehabilitation is to look after every part of ourselves.

That's the role of complementary therapies. They may seem a little strange, but they have been around for a while, and more and more people are beginning to believe that they may have some use. Ayurvedic medicine, herbal remedies, acupuncture, and various mind-body therapies are becoming more and more well-liked since they provide a more organic and complimentary method of treatment.

Consider acupuncture as an example. This is an old Chinese custom in which tiny needles are inserted into predetermined body locations. These points are like energy channels, according to Traditional Chinese Medicine, and by stimulating them you may get your qi, or vital life force, flowing in the proper direction. Although its exact mechanism of action is unknown, studies has demonstrated that it can effectively manage pain, reduce inflammation, and enhance general wellbeing.

How does this connect to hepatitis E, then? It turns out that acupuncture can really change the game in terms of symptom management. You know how hepatitis frequently coexists with symptoms like nausea, exhaustion, and stomach pain? Those nasty boys can be made better with acupuncture. As an added bonus, it can balance your energy levels and strengthen your immune system and liver. It resembles a whole bundle for recuperation and restoration.

Let's now discuss Ayurveda. The goal of this traditional Indian medical approach is to help you achieve harmony and balance inside your body. You see, illness can sneak up on you if your doshas, or energy factors, are out of balance, according to Ayurveda. Thus, the main focus of Ayurveda is determining your individual constitution and making necessary adjustments to balance things out.

What effect does this have on Hepatitis E, then? Ayurveda, however, can provide you some very astute advice on how to improve the health of your liver through dietary and lifestyle modifications. They may suggest some herbs that are proven to be effective liver defenders, such as turmeric and amla. They may even recommend that you attempt Panchakarma, a detoxification procedure, to give your liver a gentle cleaning.

We're not done yet, though. Herbal medicine plays a significant part in complementary therapies for hepatitis E. There are a plethora of herbs that have beneficial effects on the liver. Consider milk thistle as an example. It's comparable to the liver helpers super star. It can improve liver function and provide some shielding from harm. Additionally, it contains a fancy component known as silymarin, which is all about preventing oxidation and inflammation. Not to be overlooked are burdock, artichoke, and dandelion roots. All of these herbs have the ability to support your liver and aid in detoxification.

This is a crucial point to keep in mind. Your mind is just as important to holistic healing as your physical health. Managing the emotional and stress aspects of your life can significantly improve your health. Practices like yoga, mindfulness, and meditation can help you de-stress, improve your mental health, and unwind.

Let me also add that simply moving your body can have a great effect. Exercise of any form, including yoga and walking, can truly enhance your general health and promote physical healing. It all comes down to developing resilience and inner serenity even in the midst of health difficulties.

Therefore, let me inform you that on this journey to treat Hepatitis E, accepting the power of holistic healing can truly change your life. You can access millennia of knowledge and offer yourself the best chance of recovery by fusing conventional medical procedures with complementary therapies like acupuncture, Ayurveda, and herbal remedies. Additionally, you can create a mystical space for healing and recuperation when you look after your mind and your emotions.

Keep in mind that taking an active role in your own health journey is essential to holistic recovery. It's about adopting new lifestyle habits, taking care of oneself, and maintaining optimism. By doing all of that, you improve your general health and quality of life in addition to aiding in your body's healing process.

So be sure to tune in as we delve into particular comprehensive approaches to controlling Hepatitis E in the forthcoming chapters. We'll cover a wide range of topics, including healthy eating habits, effective herbal treatments, stress relief, and much more. Equipped with this comprehensive toolkit, you will own all the necessary resources to assume responsibility for your well-being and set out on a transformative path towards managing Hepatitis E.

Nourishing the Temple: The Healing Power of Nutrition

You truly need to pay close attention to your liver when managing Hepatitis E, I can assure you of that. This organ, which performs over 500 tasks to keep your body functioning properly, is very amazing. It's like the MVP of your body. It has a major role in metabolism, digestion, and detoxification. However, things start to go crazy when you have Hepatitis and it affects your liver. As inflammation progresses, the liver's ability to function is compromised. Because of this, my buddy, it's imperative that your diet focus solely on taking care of your liver.

A customised eating plan that emphasises supporting your liver's healing and nourishment is the key to effectively controlling hepatitis E. What do you know? Eating meals high in vital nutrients, antioxidants, and anti-inflammatory qualities will help you accomplish that. In addition to providing your liver with the building blocks it needs to heal itself, these superfoods also strengthen your immune system and help lower inflammation levels throughout your body. My friend, everyone wins in this scenario.

Let's now discuss the main attraction, protein. This vitamin is your liver's closest friend since it promotes the growth of new liver cells and repairs damaged ones. Furthermore, it maintains the health of your immune system, which is essential for warding off bothersome viruses and diseases. Fish, poultry, eggs, lentils, dairy products, and lean meats are good sources of protein. To be gentle on your liver, however, choose lean and low-fat foods rather than going overboard.

There's more, though! Additionally essential to the happiness and health of your liver are lipids and carbohydrates. You get the necessary energy boost from carbohydrates, which also assist control blood sugar levels. Choose complex carbohydrates, which are high in fibre and other nutrients that your liver needs, such as whole grains, fruits, and vegetables. Let's now discuss fats. My friend, they're not the enemy. Actually, in order for your liver to synthesis vital hormones and absorb all those fat-soluble vitamins, it needs them. Limit your intake of saturated and trans fats and stick to wholesome sources like avocados, nuts, seeds, and olive oil.

Oh, and don't overlook the superfoods! Packed with all the vital nutrients and antioxidants your liver loves, these bad boys are like the superheroes of the food world. Consider cruciferous veggies like broccoli and Brussels sprouts, berries, leafy greens, ginger, garlic, and turmeric. These little powerhouses will quickly aid in liver healing and boost your immune system. How delicious is this approach to assisting your body's natural healing process?

Choosing the correct meals is no longer the only step in developing a customised diet plan. You should consider food preparation techniques, cooking methods, and portion sizes. For instance, because they don't involve as much oil, grilling and baking are far healthier than frying. And make an effort to use fresh products and limit your intake of packaged and processed foods; believe me when I say that those additives and preservatives can be hard on your liver.

I have a tonne of delicious dishes that will make your path to liver health and overall wellness even more fun. They're flavorful to the extreme and nutritious at the same time! These recipes include all the foods that are good for the liver, such turmeric and garlic. Everything from a nourishing lentil soup to mouthwatering fish with quinoa and roasted vegetables is available. Prepare to indulge your taste buds while providing your body with the proper nutrition.

In summary, diet plays a critical role in the management of hepatitis E. You may assist the healing process, strengthen your immune system, and reach optimal wellbeing by realising the significance of your liver and providing it with the love and care it requires with a customised nutrition plan. Food is more than simply energy, my friend—it can be a formidable partner on your path to improved health. Accept the therapeutic potential of food and take charge of your health. You're capable!

Moving Towards Vitality: Exercise for Hepatitis E Management

I can't emphasise enough how important exercise is for controlling Hepatitis E. As a physician and health and wellness coach, I can attest to the fact that exercise can significantly improve the quality of life for individuals afflicted with Hepatitis E.

You see, in terms of our body's defence mechanism, our liver is like a superhero. It generates proteins that are essential for blood coagulation and immune system function, breaks down nutrients, and filters out contaminants. However, the liver of those who have Hepatitis E is already overworked, therefore we should take additional care of it. And exercise has a role in it.

We have shown that exercise can actually enhance liver function through a number of research. It increases circulation, breaks down stubborn lipids, and even lowers inflammation. It acts as your liver's superhero companion, helping it fight against Hepatitis E.

But exercise also strengthens your immune system, which benefits your liver. And that's quite important for people who have Hepatitis E. Hepatitis E can be prevented by our immune system, which is an amazing barrier against viruses and illnesses. Hence, regular exercise increases immune cell generation and activity, improving your body's ability to fight off those bothersome invaders.

Let's now discuss the psychological and emotional advantages of physical activity. It can be difficult to manage Hepatitis E, and it can negatively impact your mental health. Exercise can be a lifesaver in this situation. Our bodies release endorphins, which are these enchanted tiny chemicals, when we exercise. They function similarly to the "feel-good" hormones that naturally elevate you. They uplift your spirits, lessen anxiety, and possibly aid fight depression. I promise you, it will drastically improve your general quality of life.

Now that we know how crucial exercise is for treating Hepatitis E, let's get started with some personalised exercise regimens. But keep in mind that each person is different, so you should tailor your workout regimen to your personal requirements and physical limitations. A healthcare professional should always be consulted before beginning any new endeavour.

The first type of exercise is aerobic—that is, traditional cardio. It is the mainstay of any exercise programme. Low-impact activities including cycling, swimming, and walking are recommended for those with Hepatitis E. They can be adjusted to your personal exercise level and are easy on the joints.

Let's move on to the topic of strength training. Strengthening their muscles is essential for Hepatitis E patients. It enhances liver health in addition to improving physical function. As you gain strength, progressively work your way up from low weights or resistance bands. You'll be astounded by the impact it has.

Remember to be flexible and balanced! Stretching exercises help you become more flexible, which protects your joints and helps you avoid accidents. Additionally, adding balancing activities to your routine, like yoga or tai chi, can improve your stability and lower your chance of falling. They're also excellent for relieving tension and relaxing.

Lastly, we must not ignore the mind-body link. Exercise routines can benefit greatly from the incorporation of mind-body techniques such as mindfulness, meditation, and deep breathing. They support relaxation, lessen stress, and enhance mental health in general. And believe me, when it comes to coping with Hepatitis E, having a composed mind is a superpower. You'll remain upbeat and emotionally strong as a result.

Therefore, don't let adding exercise to your everyday schedule overwhelm you. Gradually increase the length and intensity of your workouts by starting small and setting realistic goals. Pay attention to your body; it is aware of your requirements. Additionally, remember to fuel yourself with a well-balanced diet that provides the nutrients you need for activity as well as maintains the function of your liver.

Exercise ultimately changes everything when it comes to treating Hepatitis E. It strengthens your immune system, facilitates better liver function, and generally improves your health. Together, let's take this trip to discover your inner strength and embrace a live that is more energetic and alive. Just keep in mind to listen to your body's signals and seek medical advice before making any significant changes to your routine. We will overcome hepatitis E because we are stronger than this.

The Mind-Body Connection: Cultivating Mindfulness

Now, let's discuss the role that mindfulness plays in healing. Really getting at the heart of the matter. Thus, mindfulness is a long-standing practise with roots in Eastern traditions. It all comes down to intentionally and impartially focusing on the here and now. We are talking about being aware of our feelings, thoughts, and physical experiences without becoming attached or alarmed. It's about embracing the present moment fully, letting go of any resistance or obsessions that may arise, and accepting what is.

Here's the issue, though: practising mindfulness isn't about wishful thinking. Actually, it has a major effect on our physical well-being. Research has demonstrated that stress and depressive feelings can adversely affect our liver, particularly in cases of hepatitis E. You see, when we're all stressed out, our bodies release stress hormones like cortisol, which interfere with the immune system and liver function. It's a very precarious situation.

But this is where practising mindfulness really helps. By lowering our stress levels, it enables our liver to resume its normal functions and maintains our general well-being. How fantastic is that?

However, mindfulness not only benefits our physical well-being but also aids in the management of our feelings and ideas related to our sickness. At times, we could experience feelings of worry, anxiety, or frustration, which exacerbates our hepatitis E symptoms and increases our stress levels. However, mindfulness allows us to notice those feelings and ideas without passing judgement. It provides us with the room to react to them in a kind and healing-promoting manner. I promise that once you get the hang of it, you'll begin building the emotional fortitude necessary to overcome all the difficulties associated with managing a chronic condition.

So how can we make mindfulness a part of our everyday lives? Fortunately for you, I own several easy-to-use yet quite effective techniques:

We started with focused breathing. Just set aside some time each day to concentrate on your breathing. As you breathe in and out, really notice how it feels. When your thoughts stray, notice how your chest rises and falls and use your breath to bring yourself back to the present.

We then practised body scan meditation. The key to this one is to set aside some time each day to thoroughly examine your entire body. Simply take note of every feature of your body without passing judgement on it. Recognize any tension or discomfort you may be experiencing and allow yourself to feel it completely. You may find areas of stress with this practise that you were unaware you possessed. After that, you can let them go and deal with them. It's really fantastic, huh?

Let's now discuss mindful eating. This one is all about giving your food your whole attention and truly enjoying every bite. Be mindful of the smells, textures, and flavours. And as you consume, pay attention to any feelings or sensations that surface. You may cultivate a more positive relationship with food and a greater appreciation for the sustenance it offers by being present throughout mealtimes.

Next is the discipline of thankfulness. Spend a few minutes every day reflecting on your blessings. It's a straightforward technique that helps you concentrate on the good things in your life. And that can help you feel less stressed, feel better emotionally, and even be healthier overall. A win-win scenario exists.

Not to mention, there was attentive movement. You can experiment with qigong, tai chi, and yoga. These exercises help you connect your mind and body in addition to increasing your physical strength and flexibility. You'll experience a level of awareness and tranquilly that you never would have believed possible by paying close attention to your breath and moving with complete awareness.

It's important for me to warn you that this mindfulness journey won't be easy. It requires dedication and repetition. Thus, begin modestly, add these attentive minutes to your everyday schedule, and then progressively increase them as you become more accustomed to them. Hey, treat yourself with kindness. Be polite and curious when you approach mindfulness. Accept and enjoy the current time to the fullest.

The amazing thing is that if you persist and truly incorporate mindfulness into your life, amazing transformations will take place. You won't be as controlled by stress. You'll be more capable of managing every obstacle that comes your way. You'll be able to ride the emotional waves without becoming overwhelmed by them. Not to mention, your liver will be eternally grateful for the reduction of stress and enhancement of your general health.

We will delve even further into the ways that mindfulness can revolutionise hepatitis E management in the upcoming chapters. We'll look at how you may incorporate it into your daily life in a variety of ways, such as your nutrition and stress management methods. I promise you that practising mindfulness will be your compass and your guide to fully managing your hepatitis E.

Stay with me, then, my friend. Let's explore the relationship between mindfulness and general health. We're going to embark on this life-changing path together to help you overcome your hepatitis E. Now is the perfect moment for empowerment and self-discovery. Are you set to go? Go now.

Unlocking the Healing Power of Nature: Herbal Remedies

You know, for ages now, humans have been using nature as a source of healing and physical care. When you think about it, it's actually sort of incredible. Herbs, or botanical medicine as some refer to it, have long been used to support general health and balance. It's sort of like a wholistic approach to self-care, you know?

Therefore, the liver suffers the most damage from Hepatitis E. Poor creature. However, some herbs are really available that can aid in the recovery process. Milk thistle is one of them. After extensive research, it was discovered that this herb possesses potent liver-protective properties. Milk thistle's silymarin, an active ingredient, functions as an antioxidant and promotes the regeneration of liver cells. What a superpower plant, you say? Studies have even demonstrated that milk thistle helps those with Hepatitis E by lowering inflammation and enhancing liver function.

Turmeric is another herb that is well worth researching. This stuff is extraordinary. It contains a substance known as curcumin, which possesses potent antioxidant and anti-inflammatory qualities. In essence, it plays a significant role in combating hepatitis E-related liver inflammation. Studies have demonstrated that curcumin can actually improve liver function and lessen indicators of liver impairment. It seems quite promising, in your opinion.

But there's still more! That material you see all over your yard, dandelion root, may also be beneficial to your liver. It turns out that liver health has long been supported by its use. These substances found in dandelion root stimulate your liver's bile production, aiding in the process of detoxification. Furthermore, it aids in digestion and the absorption of all those health-promoting elements. For your liver, it's a win-win situation.

Additionally, schisandra is a herb that has long been utilised in Traditional Chinese Medicine. It contains substances known as lignans, which have anti-inflammatory and antioxidant properties. Schisandra has been demonstrated in studies to genuinely lessen hepatitis E patients' liver inflammation and enhance their liver function. Really neat, huh?

All of these herbs can help strengthen your liver, but it's important to keep in mind that Hepatitis E is a serious illness. It's crucial to consult a physician and utilise these herbs in addition to prescribed medications. They will point you in the correct route because they are knowledgeable and capable.

And did I also mention that using herbal medicines can assist strengthen your immune system? Yes, that is true. Similar to the herb known as astragalus, which has long been utilised in Traditional Chinese Medicine due to its immune-stimulating qualities. It fortifies your body's resistance to viral illnesses, such as hepatitis E. Astragalus has been demonstrated in studies to boost antibody synthesis and immune cell function. Seems quite good, doesn't it?

The herb echinacea is another that might strengthen your immune system. It has long been used by people to cure and prevent respiratory illnesses. Furthermore, it supports the health of your liver. Interferon, a protein that functions as your immune system's super hero against viruses, is produced in greater quantities when echinacea is consumed. Therefore, echinacea can actually help lessen the intensity and duration of Hepatitis E symptoms by boosting your immune system.

Not to mention, ginseng is considered the king of adaptogens. This potent plant has the ability to alter your immune system. It stimulates the generation of cytokines, which are essential for immunological function, and increases the activity of immune cells. Thus, ginseng can boost your immune system and assist your body in fending off those pesky viral infections if you have Hepatitis E.

Now pay attention. It's important to exercise caution and ensure that the herbal medicines you're using are high-quality. Because herbal products can differ in quality, it's best to consult a trained healthcare provider who is knowledgeable about herbs. They will assist you in determining which ones are appropriate for you and ensure that the proper dosages are being used.

In summary, when it comes to treating Hepatitis E, herbal medicines are like your closest buddies. There are a tonne of incredible herbs that can help strengthen your immune system and liver function, such as ginseng, milk thistle, turmeric, dandelion root, schisandra, astragalus, and echinacea. Just keep in mind to collaborate with your medical practitioner and employ them in addition to your prescribed therapies. It's similar to discovering how to harness the force of nature to support you on your path to improved health. Take control of your health and enjoy the medicinal advantages of herbal medication now.

Medication Matters

The Antiviral Arsenal

I can't help but notice how significantly the management of viral illnesses, including the evil Hepatitis E, has changed as a result of antiviral medications. These formidable fighters operate by focusing on particular stages of the viral replication cycle, effectively saying "nay" to the virus's ambitions to proliferate and spread throughout our bodies. It's truly quite astounding. The identification and advancement of these antiviral medications has created a plethora of opportunities for the treatment of Hepatitis E, offering patients an opportunity to recover their health and quality of life. It like a ray of light amid a choppy sea.

Let's examine nucleoside analogues, a class of antiviral medicines frequently employed to treat Hepatitis E. Imagine that these medications are complete chameleons that pose as the genetic material of the virus—DNA and RNA. Clever, I realise. They totally spoil the fun for newly forming viral particles when they invade the viral genome during replication. Physicians frequently recommend the very effective nucleoside analogue ribavirin to patients suffering from either acute or chronic Hepatitis E. It has been demonstrated to inhibit viral replication and initiate a partial improvement in hepatic function.

But wait, there's still more! Protease inhibitors are another type of antiviral medications that are highly effective in the treatment of hepatitis E. These bad boys target particular enzymes that function similarly to VIPs in the processing of viral proteins. Protease inhibitors can significantly slow down viral replication and reduce the total amount of the virus in the body by sabotaging these enzymes' gears. It's equivalent to telling the virus, "You don't have VIP access!" Protease inhibitors such as boceprevir and telaprevir are demonstrating great potential in treating hepatitis E. Research has indicated that in few fortunate individuals, they not only enhance hepatic function but also decelerate the advancement of the illness.

Now hear this: one more tool in our arsenal against hepatitis E is interferon therapy. These superpower proteins are called interferons, which are produced by our body in response to viral attacks. They essentially act as the club's bouncers, preventing the spread of viruses and boosting our immunity. The preferred type of interferon for treating Hepatitis E is pegylated interferon alpha, and believe me when I say that it's revolutionary. This bad guy has demonstrated his ability to reduce the growth of viruses, improve liver health, and raise the likelihood that certain patients would see a sustained virologic response. An incredible triple threat!

Now, though, what? Researchers are not done yet. To combat hepatitis E even more potently, researchers are combining various antiviral medications to create some fascinating new concoctions. You see, the concept behind this combo therapy is to simultaneously target several viral replication cycle phases, much like in a tag-team situation. According to studies, people with chronic Hepatitis E have a far higher probability of having a sustained virologic response when they combine ribavirin and interferon alpha. These medicines seem to be saying to each other, "We're not kidding around!"

Remember that every medication has certain negative effects and the potential to interact with other medications. Because of this, before prescribing antiviral medications, medical professionals must thoroughly assess the medical history and unique circumstances of each patient. Liver function and viral load must also be closely monitored in order to ensure that the treatment is working as intended and to make necessary modifications. You have to keep an eye on it, you know?

But here's the deal, buddy: treating Hepatitis E involves more than just taking medication. Oh no, there are a tonne of holistic methods and lifestyle adjustments that can actually help. As a health and wellness coach, I'm all about giving my patients the tools they need to adopt a complete approach to managing their health. That entails focusing on diet, controlling stress, exercising, and embracing self-care practises wholeheartedly. These modest lifestyle adjustments can complement antiviral medication, improving general health and curing Hepatitis E.

The emotional and psychological rollercoaster that comes with having Hepatitis E is something we cannot ignore. Believe me when I say that getting that diagnosis can be rather overwhelming. Depression, worry, and fear can start to tag along uninvited. Giving patients the coping mechanisms and assistance they require to get through these choppy times is crucial. They are saved by counselling and psychology-related strategies, which enable them to regain their power and balance.

But there's still more. We also have complementary and alternative therapies at our disposal that are quite effective. Consider mindfulness exercises, herbal treatments, and acupuncture. These tiny jewels have demonstrated significant promise in lowering inflammation, promoting liver health, and enhancing immunological function. You know, it's like giving our bodies a little extra support.

In conclusion, the global antiviral army is growing and giving patients with hepatitis E hope. These medications, which range from protease inhibitors to nucleoside analogues, target the viral replication cycle directly and thwart the virus's objectives. Furthermore, the potency is increased to 100 when specific medications, such as ribavirin and interferon alpha, are used together. But keep in mind that treating Hepatitis E requires more than simply antiviral drugs. It involves adopting a wholistic perspective, altering our way of life, and receiving the necessary psychological assistance. Together, we can enable Hepatitis E patients to regain their health and pursue the happy, rewarding lives they so richly deserve.

The Battle of Immunity

You know, our immune system is like our own personal army when it comes to combating Hepatitis E. It serves as a line of defence against sly tiny invaders such as bacteria, viruses, and parasites. And boy, does it ever go into attack gear when it comes across the Hepatitis E virus, determined to take out the adversary and shield our frail liver from more harm.

This article discusses immune modulators and how to use them to fight Hepatitis E. These modulators are like those pharmacological versions of those covert weaponry that can strengthen our defences against the virus. They have the ability to either stimulate or repress specific immune system components, preventing virus multiplication and protecting our liver in the background.

A protein known as interferon is one of the key participants in this conflict. It is a protein that is created by our body in response to viral invasions. It can stop the Hepatitis E virus from replicating in our liver cells since it possesses potent antiviral qualities. In real life, when we have chronic Hepatitis E, doctors utilise synthetic forms of interferon, such as that sophisticated pegylated interferon-alpha, to increase our immune response. This therapy typically lasts for several months, and guess what? It has been demonstrated to be remarkably successful in getting rid of the virus in a sizable number of people.

Allow me to share with you now about another class of immune modulators that show great promise in the fight against Ebola. Interleukins are the name for these tiny organisms. These proteins are varied and have a major impact on immune response regulation. And get this: interleukin-18, in particular, is a standout among interleukins. It has been discovered to be extremely effective at increasing the production of interferon-gamma by human immune cells, hence enhancing their ability to fight viruses. Clinical trials are currently being conducted to determine the efficacy of recombinant interleukin-18 as a supplemental treatment for chronic Hepatitis E. And what's this? The preliminary findings appear quite promising.

The truth is that treating Hepatitis E involves more than just taking medication. Additionally, these naturally occurring immune modulators can help our immune system fight the virus with a little more vigour. We are discussing substances such as zinc and vitamin C, which can significantly boost our immune system, and licorice root, which has some antiviral qualities. Note that you must have a healthcare provider advising you if you plan to experiment with these natural modulators. They might not be appropriate for everyone, and they may interact with other drugs.

Imagine that the immune modulators are these valiant troops leading the charge in the fight against hepatitis E. They continuously strengthen and activate our immune system, preventing liver damage and virus multiplication. These pharmacological super heroes, which range from interleukins to interferons, are our hidden weapons that have the power to drastically alter the course of the Hepatitis E epidemic.

Hold on, buddy—not it's just about the drugs. The management of hepatitis E requires a comprehensive strategy. We discuss modifying our diets, changing our lifestyles, and even seeking out psychological treatment. As a health and wellness coach, I've come to the conclusion that the best kind of healthcare is holistic. Everything that compromises our immune system's ability to operate, such as inadequate sleep, stress, and diet, needs to be addressed. Through addressing these fundamental causes, we may fortify our barriers and enhance our general well-being.

I am aware that managing a chronic case of Hepatitis E can seem like a never-ending struggle. But we can control that virus and stop our liver from growing worse if we have the correct tools and help. It all comes down to changing one's lifestyle, taking medication interventions, and receiving psychological assistance. Through proactive management of our health and wellness, we may effectively combat Hepatitis E and create a more promising future for ourselves.

To sum up, immunity is essential in the battle against hepatitis E. We may fortify our immune response and shield our fragile liver from further harm by using immune modulators, both herbal and pharmaceutical. These immune modulators, which range from interleukins to interferons, are the weapons in our armoury that are prepared to change the course of the fight against hepatitis E. However, we must not overlook the wider picture. The key is to adopt a holistic strategy by changing your lifestyle, obtaining the proper diet, and locating support. With all of these components in place, we can enhance our results and give those impacted by hepatitis E a better future.

Navigating Side Effects

Now that we have that out of the way, let's discuss some of the less than enjoyable aspects of taking hepatitis E medicine. Gastrointestinal issues are one thing you may encounter. They can be a tremendous pain in the, well, you know where, I promise. Constipation, diarrhoea, vomiting, and nausea can all make an appearance. It's undoubtedly difficult and can seriously impair your general wellbeing. But fear not—these adverse effects may be controlled. Start by keeping an eye on your diet. Stick to smaller, more frequent meals that are easy to digest; heavy or oily foods will only make matters worse. Remember to remain hydrated as well! To prevent becoming dehydrated, make sure you're receiving enough fluids. Do not hesitate to seek professional help from your healthcare practitioner if things are becoming out of control or if they are not going away.

Skin responses are another possible adverse effect. And believe me when I say that these responses may really get under your skin. They are difficult to ignore and might manifest as redness, irritation, or rashes. So, be sure to notify your healthcare professional as soon as you observe any changes in your skin. They are able to determine whether the issue is caused by your medication or by anything else. They might be armed with ointments or creams to help with these skin problems. Hey, they may even need to modify your prescription regimen.

Oh, and let's not overlook the possibility of weakness and exhaustion during Hepatitis E therapy. What a complete buzzkill, don't you think? Your daily tasks may begin to feel like an ascent of Mount Everest. But don't worry, buddy. Here, your greatest option will be to prioritise getting enough sleep and relaxing. Give yourself permission to take pauses when necessary and pay attention to your body. Additionally, deep breathing exercises, meditation, and mild exercise may be your best bet for boosting your energy and warding off exhaustion. However, don't be afraid to tell your healthcare physician if the exhaustion is persistent or if it's keeping you down for what seems like forever. To assist you combat the tiredness monster, they might need to make adjustments to your prescription schedule or provide you with some extra advice.

This one is worth mentioning even though it's not as common. hair fall. Yes, it is possible for some patients receiving treatment for hepatitis E to have it. And let's face it, having your hair cut can seriously damage your confidence and sense of self. Consult your healthcare professional if you begin to notice that your hair is shouting "adios." They can look into whether the reason for the hair loss is something else entirely, or if it's connected to your medicine. They can even recommend vitamins that could aid in the robust, healthy regrowth of your hair. They might also have some hair care advice.

Now, everyone, hold on tight—we're not quite done yet. While receiving therapy for hepatitis E, some patients may also have mood swings and emotional ups and downs. Yes, excellent stuff. It could feel like you're riding a rollercoaster, with moments of happiness followed by sadness and then who knows what. Acknowledging and sharing these changes with your healthcare physician is crucial. They can suggest counselling or therapy to assist you get through the difficult emotional times. In certain instances, they may need to modify your medication to help you regain emotional equilibrium.

This is the point where we explore the world of our blood friends. Medication for hepatitis E has occasionally been observed to interfere with our blood values. Red blood cell, white blood cell, and platelet counts can all become unstable. For this reason, during treatment, routine blood tests are essential. Your healthcare practitioner is the one with all the answers if something strange appears. To restore optimal blood quality, they may need to modify your medication or administer extra treatments.

Finally, and most definitely not least, neurological and cognitive symptoms are the rarest of the rare. Yes, I realise that sounds like something from a science fiction film, but really does happen. Difficulties focusing, memory issues, confusion, and even seizures may knock on your door. In the event that this occurs, visit your healthcare physician right away rather than waiting for an invitation. To determine the best course of action, they will conduct a complete review. It could entail changing your prescription regimen or, for a more thorough evaluation, consulting a neurologist.

That concludes our journey through the adverse effects of treatment for hepatitis E. Although it's not the most glamorous path, we must deal with it anyway. It's important to recognise these possible adverse effects and address them as soon as possible. Communicate openly and honestly with your healthcare practitioner. They are available to support you during your highs and lows. We can defeat Hepatitis E together and provide a seamless recuperation for you.

Beyond Medication: Holistic Approaches

Dietary Changes

Now let's discuss using food's healing properties to manage Hepatitis E. Having worked as a medical practitioner as well as a health and wellness coach, I am aware of how crucial it is to customise diets to meet the specific needs of every individual. Although there isn't a diet designed specifically for Hepatitis E, there are adjustments we can do to assist manage symptoms and promote liver recovery.

Above all, we must abstain from alcohol like the plague. As much as I understand how alluring a glass of wine might be after a long day, alcohol consumption while having Hepatitis E is like buying a one-way ticket to liver trouble. So, let's abstain from alcohol while receiving therapy and recovering, shall we?

Let's now discuss eating a balanced diet. Our goal is to consume more fruits, vegetables, whole grains, lean proteins, and low amounts of fat. These nutritional powerhouses provide our systems with the antioxidants and nutrients they require to fend against infections and support the regeneration and repair of our liver cells. Not to mention the importance of minerals like magnesium and zinc, as well as vitamins B, C, and E; they are our liver's super healers on the side.

And let's not overlook how crucial it is to maintain proper hydration. Water is our hidden weapon in this situation because it keeps our digestion going smoothly and helps flush away those terrible poisons. Staying hydrated is like giving our body an internal high five, especially for warriors against Hepatitis E.

Stress Management Techniques

Are you under stress? You're not alone, so don't worry. And you know what? The symptoms of hepatitis E can worsen while under stress. So let's put an end to tension and welcome the healing energy of Zen.

Exercises involving deep breathing are one trick up our sleeves. Inhale deeply, and then exhale gradually. Sensation that? We are teaching our bodies to relax when we pay attention to our breath. It's similar to turning on the neurological system's relaxation mode by flipping a switch. Say goodbye to tension and hello to calm.

A further method for reducing stress is mindfulness meditation. This one is all about finding our centre of peace and accepting the moment as it is. We can pay attention to our breathing, our body's sensations, or even a single object. While doing this, we're allowing ideas to come and go without passing judgement, much like clouds. It's similar to going on a tranquil mental vacation to an island.

Furthermore, physical activity is fantastic for reducing stress. Choose between a pleasant jog, yoga, or tai chi! It not only improves our fitness, lifts our spirits, and gives us more energy, but it also helps us manage our stress levels. There is win-win.

Sleep and Rest

For a moment, let's cuddle up and discuss sleep and relaxation. You are aware of the significance of restful sleep for the healing process, don't you? Well, for all of us Hepatitis E warriors, it's very necessary.

Let's establish a calming bedtime ritual to guarantee we obtain the sleep of our dreams. It could be as easy as curling up with a book, having a warm bath, or turning on some calming music. To enable us to fall asleep and dream, it is important to provide a calm and distraction-free sleeping environment.

But there's still more! We must remember to obtain enough sleep during the day as well. This could entail incorporating quick pauses into our tasks, learning some relaxation methods, or even fitting in a quick power sleep. Recall that in order for our bodies to repair and regenerate, they require care.

Complementary Therapies

Complementary therapies are where things start to get interesting. These bad boys can make us feel like superheroes and give our bodies an extra push in the healing department.

Acupuncture is one such approach. Yes, those tiny needles may seem scary, but they really do have magical powers. They cause the release of endorphins, which function as the body's own endogenous analgesics. Furthermore, acupuncture can strengthen our immune system and enhance liver function in the fight against hepatitis E. Talk about the team's victory.

Next up is herbal medicine. With good cause, this one has been around for a very long time. Herbs that are known to assist liver function and detoxification include milk thistle, dandelion, and turmeric. Hey, take note: in order to reap the greatest and safest advantages from these puppies, always seek the advice of a licenced herbal medicine practitioner.

Have you ever tried getting a massage? It's the art of relaxing, to put it simply. Our entire body exhales in relaxation when the tension in our muscles is released. And let's not overlook aromatherapy, either. The rich aromas of essential oils can soothe, uplift, and promote our overall wellbeing. They're like a spa day for our emotions.

Emotional Support

Now that we have discussed the emotional aspects of having hepatitis E, let's move on. It's difficult, and our emotions might run amok. For this reason, we require a support structure to guide us through those challenging situations.

My focus in my profession is on offering psychological treatments, counselling, and emotional support. Together, we can recognise harmful thought patterns, break free from them, and create constructive coping mechanisms. And you know what? Seeking out genuine understanding from friends, family, and support groups can make a world of difference.

There you have it: a comprehensive strategy for treating Hepatitis E. We have everything we need to take charge of our recovery process, including altering our food, controlling our stress levels, putting rest and sleep first, investigating complementary therapies, and attending to our mental wellbeing. It's time to maximise our health and let our inner warrior out! Let's get started!

The Future of Hepatitis E Treatment

Allow me to share with you the exciting adventure that lies ahead for the treatment of hepatitis E. The medical community is seeing a tsunami of discoveries, breakthroughs, and new opportunities that are upending the status quo. This narrative will have you on the edge of your seat, so hold on tight.

Let's talk about these newly developed antiviral treatments first. Researchers have made some astounding discoveries in recent years that could revolutionise the way Hepatitis E is treated. Direct-acting antiviral agents (DAAs) are fancy-sounding medications that target the core of the virus. These tiny bad boys are preventing the virus from replicating, and I have to say that the results are very amazing. Imagine a scenario where clinical trials are transforming the medical community by demonstrating exceptional viral clearance rates and bettering the prognosis of individuals suffering from chronic Hepatitis E.

Folks, that's not all. Seize your opportunity, as we are about to explore a whole new realm of combination medicines. Things start to get extremely exciting at this point. Several antiviral medications are being added to the mix in an effort to increase therapeutic efficacy. These researchers are outwitting the virus and giving it a severe beating by mixing various medications that attack it in different ways. Doesn't that seem like something from a science fiction film? Preliminary research is yielding some encouraging findings, including shorter treatment durations and increased rates of sustained virologic response. Things are starting to get better for everyone suffering with hepatitis E, as if they have finally figured out the code.

Hold on for a moment. I have one more astounding revelation for you. Get ready to explore the realm of immunity modulators. These bad boys aren't content to just take direct aim at the infection.

Oh no, they have more ambitious ambitions. Their goal is to strengthen the body's defences against the virus and assist it in doing so. They are creating medications that boost the immune system in addition to taking aim at the infection. My friends, this entails more than just getting rid of the virus. It entails offering sustained protection against Hepatitis E and avoiding reinfection. That is what I refer to as a double whammy.

But there's still more. These scientists are delving further into the investigation of host-targeted treatments. They're attempting to solve the mystery of what causes this illness to spread, much like detectives. They are thwarting the virus's malicious intentions and lessening its effects on the liver by focusing on particular cellular functions that it grabs onto. This novel strategy has the potential to avert problems and challenge the status quo of hepatitis E.

Let's now discuss customised medicine. This is the point at which things get genuinely personal. Thanks to numerous sophisticated developments in genetics and molecular diagnostics, medical professionals are now able to design individualised therapy regimens. Based on your genetic profile, they will be able to determine if you are more susceptible to a severe illness or whether you will respond exceptionally well to a particular treatment. It's similar to having a personal physician who is aware of your particular needs. My friends, we're done with treating everyone the same way. It's all about you and what makes you special.

And you know what? The future is arrived, and with it, some very magical technological advancements. My friends, telemedicine is altering the rules. Envision always having your physician at your disposal, no matter where you are. They can keep an eye on you from a distance, educate you, and modify your treatment plan. It's like to carrying about a medical superhero. It not only increases accessibility to healthcare but also helps you stay motivated and on course with your treatment. This is the way that Hepatitis E will be managed in the future, and you can do it all from the comfort of your own home.

Hey, let's not overlook the importance of prevention. Even while these treatments are amazing, our primary goal should still be to prevent Hepatitis E before it even arises. In certain regions of the globe, vaccination campaigns have shown to be extremely successful. Thus, let us continue our research and make investments to create even more effective vaccinations. Since eradicating new infections and controlling hepatitis E worldwide are the ultimate goals.

Thus, dear friends, it appears that there is hope for the cure of hepatitis E. We're getting closer to a time when Hepatitis E is not a public health issue thanks to all these new treatments, tailored medicine, and technology advancements. The field of Hepatitis E research is advancing at a rapid pace, and I am confident that working together, we can defeat this illness and create a better future. Settle in, people. We're in for an incredible journey.

Navigating Nutrition

The Power of Nutrient-Rich Foods

Our liver is quite amazing, you know. It's like this mega organ that controls so many vital bodily functions, including metabolism, hormone balance, and detoxification. However, providing it with extra care through a healthy diet becomes even more crucial when it's being attacked by something like Hepatitis E. Really, when you think about it, our liver requires the same nutrients that we do to stay healthy.

Now, let's explore the realm of vitamins that are essential for liver health. Let's start with vitamin A. This super vitamin supports and strengthens our liver, acting as a kind of cheerleader for it. This vitamin is present in foods such as sweet potatoes, carrots, and some very leafy greens like kale and spinach. Thus, add some of these delectables to your next salad or stir-fry and give your liver a high five.

Alright, let's meet Vitamin E, another vitamin that loves our livers. This bad boy intervenes to shield our liver cells from harm caused by those bothersome free radicals, acting as if he were a superhero antioxidant. Vitamin E can be found lurking in foods such as seeds, almonds, and vegetable oils. You know those walnuts or almonds you like to nibble on? They defend the health of your liver like tiny Vitamin E superheroes. Remember that pumpkin seeds are also very powerful.

But really, vitamins aren't the only thing. Minerals are similar to the ancillary components that our liver need. Selenium is a superstar mineral that has been shown to have strong antioxidant properties and protect our liver cells from damage. Selenium is abundant in foods including eggs, shellfish, and Brazil nuts. So give your liver a pat on the back and enjoy some Brazil nuts, seafood, or a delicious omelette.

Let's now discuss antioxidants, another set of heroes. These folks are comparable to the emergency responders who head to the site of oxidative stress and inflammation in the liver. And they do a fantastic job of putting out the fires. Berries: Raspberries, blueberries, and strawberries are good sources of antioxidants. I don't know about you, but I adore eating a large bowl of oats topped with a few of these vibrant jewels to start my day. It makes my liver feel like it's being celebrated.

And let's not overlook leafy greens. These guys clean up toxins and aid in the liver's detoxification process; they're like the housekeepers of our bodies. Swiss chard, spinach, and kale are all superfoods in and of themselves. You may stir-fry them or sauté them with little garlic and olive oil. There are countless methods to incorporate more leafy greens into your diet.

The problem is that specific nutrients aren't the only consideration. It concerns the entire bundle. Whole foods are like our liver's best support system; examples include quinoa, brown rice, lentils, and chickpeas. They include fibre, vitamins, minerals, and a host of other nutrients that our liver requires to function properly. Thus, be sure to fill your plate with these healthful items.

And come on, let's cook in a healthful manner. The good guys of cooking techniques include steaming, baking, and grilling since they help us retain the nutrients in our food. Conversely, not so much when it comes to fries. So let's avoid deep frying and stick to cooking techniques that preserve nutritional value.

Here's a quick advice for you: eat mindfully. It functions similarly to a covert weapon, improving our ability to absorb and process nutrients. Thus, chew your meal thoroughly, give each bite a lot of attention, and pay attention to your body's cues about hunger and fullness. You can help your liver's healing process and show your body some love during mealtimes by being mindful and in the moment.

You know, adding these nutrient-dense foods to your regular diet offers you the opportunity to experience a whole new range of tastes and sensations in addition to helping you manage your Hepatitis E. The options are unlimited, ranging from colourful fruits and vegetables to filling grains and proteins. So use your imagination in the kitchen. Experiment with various herbs and spices. Prepare dishes that are not only incredibly tasty but also healthy for your liver.

Let the power of nutrient-rich foods be your beacon of guidance as you set out on this path to manage Hepatitis E. Accept the flavours and colours they provide, and observe how they improve your general state of well-being. You are providing your body with nourishment with every bite, aiding in the healing process of your liver, and making significant progress toward full control of your Hepatitis E. You can do this!

Unmasking the Hidden Culprits

It's amazing to consider how integrated processed foods have gotten into our daily lives. Well, I understand. We're constantly searching for something nice and quick to eat. The problem is that all those easy snacks we adore eating have a cost: our poor health. Were you aware of the damage that these processed foods can do to our livers? Yes, they have enough sodium in them to last a lifetime along with all these artificial additives and preservatives. What is the result of that? It seriously messes with our bodies. Man, our livers take a serious hit. They are in charge of handling all the poisons that are directed towards us, but when they are overloaded with this garbage, they become overwhelmed. That's when everything goes wrong and our livers suffer greatly.

However, do you know what's even worse? All those sugar-filled beverages that we are consuming excessively. They really are everywhere! All of them, from pricey energy drinks to soda, are full of added sugars and empty calories. Like, this is like a huge amount of sugar. It not only causes weight gain and increases our chance of developing conditions like diabetes, but it also severely strains our livers. Our livers are similar to sugar factories, you see. They are meant to convert all of the sugar we eat into energy that our systems can utilise. However, when we consume sugar-filled beverages in large quantities, our livers find it difficult to keep up. What do you think happens next? Fat begins to accumulate in our hepatic cells, causing havoc throughout. Non-alcoholic fatty liver disease is a serious condition. It's essentially a stepping stone to more serious liver conditions, and believe me when I say that it exacerbates the Hepatitis E symptoms.

Let's talk about those bad fats now. They resemble the sinister stepmothers of liver function. All of those delicious baked items, processed snacks, and fried foods sneakily include these trans and saturated fats. They taste great, I know, but they're like a liver-exploding time bomb. They inflame the body as if it were their own. The worst aspect, too? They're seriously interfering with our liver function, not simply causing us to put on weight and become blobs. You see, the function that our livers do is to break down and process lipids so that our bodies can use them as fuel. When we consume a reasonable amount of healthy fats, we're alright, but when we overindulge in bad fats, our livers become overworked. When they feel as though they are drowning in fatty acids, hepatic steatosis begins to manifest. It not only impairs the function of our livers, but it also creates a gateway to more severe liver illnesses.

Hey, though, don't worry. My friend, there's always a way out. You just must be an expert at interpreting those deceptive nutrition labels. Food makers have a tendency to mislead us into believing that their products are nutritious when in reality they are not. We are duped when they slap on labels that declare something to be "natural" or "low-fat." The fact is, though, that those items still tend to be loaded with harmful fats, artificial junk, and hidden sugars. Take some time to truly comprehend what those nutrition labels are trying to tell you the next time you're at the grocery store. After all, we're talking about the condition of your liver.

Not to be overlooked is the packaging. It feels so much like a trap. We get the impression that those foods are authentic because of their utilisation of eye-catching designs and vivid colours. But my friend, don't fall for it. They're merely manipulating us mentally. So, you know, we need to be wise shoppers. Remain knowledgeable and identify the unhealthy foods concealed by attractive packaging. They cannot prevail. Our livers are worthy of more.

I have to tell you that in the fight against Hepatitis E, information truly is power. It all comes down to staying away from these processed meals, sweetened beverages, and bad fats. You're giving your liver a better chance by doing that. By doing so, you're lowering inflammation, improving the symptoms, and laying the groundwork for a healthier liver and a more promising future. It is now the ideal moment to adopt a diet rich in complete, unprocessed foods, such as fruits, vegetables, lean meats, and healthy fats. Your liver is aching for those nutrients, guy. Additionally, remember to move and drink plenty of water. Engaging in physical activity is akin to giving your liver a small present that keeps it healthy and helps you feel your best.

So, my friend, pay attention. We'll go into more detail on strategies to help your liver mend and improve your general health in the upcoming chapter. We'll discuss the benefits of herbal medicines and the potency of antioxidants, providing you with all the information you need to take charge of your Hepatitis E journey. Because, as you may recall, you possess the ability to restore your health and unleash the healing powers of your liver. It's all up to you.

The Art of Meal Planning

As a physician and health and wellness consultant, I can honestly say that meal planning has brought about some amazing changes in people's lives. Choosing what to eat for breakfast, lunch, and supper is only one step in a lengthy process that takes into account your needs, tastes, and health objectives. And meal planning becomes even more important for managing Hepatitis E. I am referring to the significant influence that adequate diet can have on maintaining liver function and averting additional harm. You might think of it as donning a superhero costume to help your liver do its magic and keep you feeling your best.

You may be asking, then, how one even begins to learn the skill of meal planning. Alright, let us dissect it together, step by step.

Assess Your Goals and Needs

Prior to starting the meal planning process, stop, think about what you want to accomplish. Do you want to get in better shape overall, keep your weight in check, or lose weight? Your meal planning adventure will go lot more smoothly if you know what your goals are. Furthermore, remember to take into account any dietary limitations or allergies you may have. When looking for recipes and ingredients, we need to take into account if you have a gluten or lactose intolerance.

Create a Balanced Menu

A well-balanced diet hits all the proper notes for your body, much like a symphony of flavours and nutrients. To keep things interesting and lively, start by giving each day of the week a theme, such as Meatless Monday or Fish Friday. In this manner, your plate will have a diversity of ingredients and you won't become tired of the same foods.

Let's talk about protein now. Your go-to foods should include lean meats, fish, poultry, beans, and legumes. Aim for a minimum of one serving of protein with every meal to maintain the health of your muscles and liver.

Remember to include fruits and vegetables on your meal; they are like the vibrant sidekicks. Brimming with fibre and antioxidants, they do wonders for your liver and general well-being.

Hey, don't forget to eat entire grains and good fats. Choose whole grain products such as pasta, bread, rice, and cereals; also, include nuts, seeds, avocados, and olive oil as healthy sources of fat. Inflammation will decrease and your heart will appreciate it.

Incorporate Liver-Friendly Ingredients

We are now moving this meal planning process to a new level. It's time to unleash the liver-friendly components' hidden weapon. According to research, your liver can benefit greatly from a few certain foods and nutrients that lower inflammation and aid in the detoxification process.

Take a look at this: turmeric is a great spice that battles inflammation like a pro. It contains a substance known as curcumin, which shields your liver from a variety of stresses.

Not to be overlooked are the cruciferous vegetables, such as cauliflower posse, Brussels sprouts, and broccoli. These guys are a powerful source of sulphur compounds and antioxidants that support liver detoxification and maintain your liver in combat mode.

Berries, green tea, garlic, and fatty seafood like salmon are also included. Therefore, don't be scared to play around with flavours and spices to make delicious meals that are also really healthy for your liver.

Plan Ahead and Prep

I'm going to get right to the point, my friend. Meal planning is more than just choosing what to eat; it's also about organising your schedule and cooking like a pro. This is the magic ingredient that keeps you on the right track by removing stress and time restrictions.

The task at hand is to schedule a dedicated period of time each week for organising and preparing meals. Now is the time to look for recipes, make a list of things to buy, and prepare those ingredients. I promise that having everything you need close at hand eliminates the need for poor eating habits and late-night munching.

Imagine this: batch cooking. For later consumption, cook some meals in bigger quantities and split them into individual servings. For those hectic days when you're simply not in the mood to cook, you may even freeze them. Simple as pie, huh?

Be Flexible and Enjoy the Process

You've reached the final stage, my friend. And that one is revolutionary. While having a strategy is undoubtedly necessary, it's as important to be adaptable and enjoy the process. Organizing meals shouldn't ever feel like a chore or a punishment. It's about appreciating the impact food has on your well-being, connecting with the food you eat, and feeding your soul just as much as your body.

So go ahead and try those new dishes, taste other flavours, and allow yourself to indulge in a treat now and then. The key to both full Hepatitis E management and a lifetime of health and wellbeing is meal planning. Take charge of your diet from now on, and show your liver the respect it deserves. I promise that your liver will be thanking you with a glass of purifying green juice.

Supercharged Smoothies and Juices

Hi everyone! Let's discuss liver health and the significant impact that diet has on our health. You see, there's a clear correlation between our nutrition and the health of our organs, with our livers receiving special attention. This amazing organ performs a multitude of functions for us, including blood sugar regulation, bile assisting in digestion, detoxification of our systems, and the breakdown of hazardous substances. Giving it the assistance it requires is therefore essential.

Incorporating supercharged juices and smoothies into your regular routine is one way to do that. Rich in vital nutrients, antioxidants, and enzymes that support liver detoxification and enhance overall function, these potent elixirs are loaded with potency. The best thing, though? They taste great in addition to being healthy.

The bright green smoothies are one kind that is very popular among supercharged smoothies. These beauties are packed full of leafy greens that are believed to cleanse the liver, such parsley, kale, and spinach. These greens' chlorophyll aids in detoxifying your liver by removing poisons from it. But there's still more! By including superfoods like spirulina, chlorella, or wheatgrass, you can kick it up a notch. These fellas are loaded with antioxidants, vitamins, and minerals to support the health and happiness of your liver.

We've got you covered if you're more of a fruit person. That's berries all the way! Antioxidants, vitamins, and fibre from blueberries, strawberries, raspberries, and blackberries shield your liver from oxidative stress. These little creatures are your liver's best pals, I promise. Add some turmeric, ginger, or cinnamon to enhance the antioxidant content to make things even better. Curcumin, a potent chemical found in turmeric, reduces inflammation, while ginger calms and cinnamon regulates blood sugar.

Making your own supercharged juices and smoothies allows you to customise them to your liver's exact requirements, which is the beauty of it all. You can play around to target certain liver processes or take care of any underlying medical conditions. For example, beets are a great ally if you want to promote detoxification. They have this amazing antioxidant called betalain, which promotes bile flow and liver detoxification.

And believe me when I say that creating these hypercharged items is an entirely unique experience. It's quite another to gather the components, combine them, and then enjoy the finished product—the that's therapeutic part. It's a joyful and fulfilling mindful exercise that allows you to appreciate the flavours and brilliant colours that nourish your body. Furthermore, this procedure promotes general well-being in addition to the nutrients.

As a physician and health and wellness coach, I have seen firsthand how supercharged smoothies and juices affect my hepatitis E patients. Their wellbeing has significantly improved when these drinks are included in a comprehensive plan for controlling the illness. Their general health improved, their energy levels rose, and their liver function improved.

So, get enthusiastic if you're prepared to set out on a delectable trip towards the best possible liver health! You're about to discover an entire universe of enhanced smoothie and juice creations. There is something for everyone, from antioxidant-rich fruit elixirs to cool green mixtures. So grab that blender and let's give your liver a liquid-rich boost to help it heal. To your health, cheers!

The Healing Symphony of Herbs and Spices

As a physician and health and wellness coach, I must admit that I am a huge proponent of holistic medicine and wellbeing. You know, it's not only about prescription drugs and medical procedures. Certain natural therapies are available that can significantly accelerate the healing process. That's where spices and herbs come into play, my friend.

These tiny miracles have been utilised for their therapeutic qualities for ages in a variety of cultures. And you know what? Tradition has finally been surpassed by science. It appears that these spices and herbs have a plethora of health benefits! They have the potential to be quite beneficial, particularly in the management of Hepatitis E.

Shall we begin with turmeric? Imagine a brilliant yellow spice that is added to curry recipes. Turmeric is that! This bad boy contains a substance known as curcumin. And let me tell you, curcumin is a powerful anti-inflammatory and liver-protecting substance. It even increases the generation of bile, which aids in digestion and maintains optimal liver function. Add some turmeric to your soup, curry, or even to make golden milk. Your liver will be appreciative!

Let's go on to ginger. This material is very timeless, my friend. Ginger has been used for ages to treat digestive issues of many types and to settle unsettled stomachs. And you know what? It is quite effective for Hepatitis E patients. Bloating, pain in the stomach, and nausea? Ginger is on top of things. Fresh ginger can be sprinkled on food or used to drinks and smoothies. A tiny bit of ginger goes a long way.

Shall we add some cinnamon to liven things up? This one offers numerous health advantages in addition to enhancing the taste and warmth of your food. For your liver, cinnamon is like a superpower. It defends the liver, reduces inflammation, and even aids in blood sugar regulation. And believe me when I say that this last bit is critical for those with Hepatitis E since the infection interferes with the creation of insulin. Add a dash of cinnamon to your roasted vegetables, blend it into your smoothies, or stir it into your daily porridge. I promise it will revolutionise the game.

Let's now discuss milk thistle. This plant has been used for ages to help detoxification and liver function. It contains a substance known as silymarin, which possesses numerous anti-inflammatory and antioxidant properties. How wonderful it is to preserve and regenerate liver cells! By increasing the synthesis of glutathione, milk thistle can also aid in liver detoxification. And believe me when I say that glutathione acts as your body's small shield against toxic substances. You can relax with a cup of milk thistle tea or buy milk thistle supplements. However, always with your physician before starting any new regimen.

Let me finally inform you about the root dandelion. Yes, I understand that you consider it to be an obtrusive weed, but guess what? In fact, it has a wealth of medicinal qualities, particularly for liver health. This stuff, my friend, is amazing. Its abundance of minerals and antioxidants supports and aids in the detoxification of your liver. In addition, dandelion root stimulates the formation of bile, which helps the liver eliminate waste and regulates digestion. Use the leaves in your salads or enjoy some dandelion root tea. You'll be loved by your liver for it.

Now, I want you to keep in mind that although spices and herbs are wonderful, they cannot take the place of prescription drugs or medical treatments. Consult a healthcare professional before making any significant decisions. My friend, they'll provide you with the best guidance depending on your particular demands.

In summary, the universe of herbs and spices is similar to a liver-healing symphony. These natural medicines, which include the calming properties of ginger, the potency of turmeric, and the detoxifying properties of milk thistle and dandelion root, can truly enhance medical interventions and hasten the healing process. Therefore, my friend, get inventive in the kitchen. Try different flavours. For some amazing grilled chicken, combine garlic, ginger, and turmeric in a marinade. Or you may add a dash of nutmeg and cinnamon to your roasted sweet potatoes to make them more flavorful. Elevate your meals and allow these restorative components to do their job as you manage your Hepatitis E.

Mind Over Matter

The Hidden Power of the Mind

What's wild, you know? It turns out that our physical health is greatly influenced by our ideas and feelings. For example, our body sets out a stress alarm when we experience stress or low mood. And believe me when I say that this alert sets off a cascade of stress chemicals, including cortisol, which can do nothing more than impair immunity and make it much more difficult for the body to fight off illnesses like hepatitis E. Crazy, you say?

On the other hand, having a positive outlook and feeling good about ourselves truly improves our general state of wellbeing. I'm not kidding when I say that research indicates those with cheerful and upbeat attitudes typically have healthier bodies and recover from ailments more quickly. It's as if our minds possess a superpower that enables us to recover from and resist illnesses like hepatitis E.

So how can we access this latent mental power? First and foremost, we need to be conscious of our ideas and feelings. We must be aware of the bodily effects they have on us as well as how they impact our general wellbeing. After we've mastered that, we can deliberately focus on nurturing those feelings of well-being and embracing a perspective that centres upon taking control of our recovery process.

A nice technique to attract good energy is to cultivate thankfulness. I mean to say that we should recognise and value the small things in life that bring us joy. Though it may sound corny, studies have shown that thankfulness can strengthen our immune systems, improve our mental health, and promote physical healing. So why not attempt it? Perhaps incorporating a daily appreciation practise into our routine can keep us optimistic and aid our body's defence against Hepatitis E.

Imagine this for a moment: visualising. By using our imagination, we can visualise ourselves in perfect health, our immune systems destroying any illness that threatens us. It's similar to rewriting our thoughts and beliefs about resilience and healing into our subconscious. You have to admit, that is just astounding.

The shocking thing is that controlling Hepatitis E with mental power involves more than just looking after our bodily health. Zooming out, we also need to consider our mental, emotional, and spiritual health. This is the role of self-care. It's about taking care of our mind, body, and soul—not it's just about face masks and bubble baths. such as journaling, deep breathing, meditation, and other beneficial practises. And you know what? Establishing a self-care regimen truly helps our bodies heal and maintains our mental health.

Hold on now. I want to be really clear about something. Using mental techniques to manage Hepatitis E does not imply forgoing medical care. Not in a manner. It all comes down to enhancing the efficacy of conventional medical techniques by collaborating with them. It's important to address our health and wellbeing holistically to improve our chances of recovery and ensure our long-term health.

In summary, the ability to harness the hidden power of the mind can significantly transform the management of Hepatitis E. We may use the power of our ideas, emotions, and physical health to heal, recover, and live our best lives when we recognise this link. By implementing techniques such as self-care, visualisation, and appreciation, we may unleash our potential and design a strategy to eradicate Hepatitis E. You can do this. Beyond Hepatitis E, you possess the ability to empower your own healing process and live a more radiant life.

Unraveling the Stress-Disease Connection

You know, they say that hepatitis E isn't primarily caused by stress. Nope, it's actually spread by tainted water, particularly in areas where sanitary conditions are subpar. The twist is that stress escalates the situation, exacerbating the symptoms and delaying the healing process. Studies reveal that individuals with long-term stress are more vulnerable to Hepatitis E and require more time to recover than those with stress-reduction strategies.

Let me explain it to you now: there is a complex dance going on between stress and illness that involves our mind, body, and immune system. Our body's stress reaction kicks in when stress interrupts the party, releasing a hopscotch of hormones including cortisol and adrenaline. These hormones can save your life in an emergency, but if stress persists for an extended period of time, they can cause serious damage. Stress hormones have a detrimental effect on our immune system, making us vulnerable to infections and prolonging diseases like hepatitis E.

The bottom line is that stress affects not just our immune system but also our behaviour and decision-making. We may go for the bottle more frequently or turn to junk food treatment when stress gets the better of us. Not good news for our liver or our recuperation. Furthermore, stress can weaken our immune systems, spoil our beautiful sleep, and exacerbate Hepatitis E symptoms including weariness and stomach ache.

But fear not, my companion. This stress storm and its effect on hepatitis E can be avoided. We must apply some efficient stress-reduction tactics and strategies in order to target stress where it hurts. Let's examine a couple of them:

First up is mindfulness meditation, which is just a fancy way of saying that we should concentrate on the here and now, without passing judgement. It turns out that this exercise helps lower stress levels, improve our emotional health, and strengthen our immune system. It resembles constructing a barrier to keep pressures out.

There's heavy breathing after that. Who knew that relieving stress with a few deep breaths could have such a magical effect? Exercises involving deep breathing, such as belly breathing, switch on the body's relaxation response and assist in regulating stress chemicals. Breathing exercises can greatly reduce stress and improve our general state of well-being.

Another undiscovered weapon in the fight against stress is movement. Regular physical activity, whether it be a jog, a yoga session, or a stroll in the park, can drastically reduce stress and strengthen our immune system. Exercise keeps our liver functioning properly and releases endorphins, those feel-good chemicals. It feels like a double whammy that relieves stress.

Let's talk about food now. For the purpose of supporting our liver and maintaining a robust immune system, eating a healthy diet is crucial. A diet rich in fruits, vegetables, lean proteins, and whole grains that is well-balanced is like having the winning ticket to a healthy body. Additionally, avoid processed foods, too much sugar, and alcohol as they will only exacerbate liver stress and impede the healing process.

However, we must not overlook beauty sleep. Restful sleep is vital for both our body and mind. However, stress has a way of messing it up, making it difficult to fall asleep or keep those Z's flowing. Therefore, we need to develop healthy sleeping habits, such as following a schedule, establishing a nightly ritual, and transforming our bedroom into a haven. I promise you that getting more sleep boosts your immunity and expedites your recuperation from hepatitis E.

Hey, we're not doing this by ourselves. Having a strong support network of family, friends, and medical professionals around us may do wonders for reducing stress and improving our general wellbeing. By talking to others who have experienced similar things, connecting with like-minded individuals, and sharing our concerns, we may overcome Hepatitis E with courage and strength.

Not to mention, there are numerous stress-reduction techniques we might employ. It's worth trying progressive muscle relaxation, visualisation exercises, aromatherapy, and journaling. It's similar to opening a grab bag full of stressors. The secret is figuring out what works best for us and incorporating these methods into our everyday lives.

So, my friend, you can take control of your physical and emotional health if you have these stress-reduction techniques in your back pocket. Recall that stress management is a continuous process, so maintain these methods and reap their rewards. Bid farewell to stress's cunning role in the development of hepatitis E. Gain control, overcome your stress, and make progress toward a better, healthier future.

The Emotion Epidemic

Receiving the news that you have Hepatitis E feels like a kick to the stomach. Anxiety and fear come over you like a tidal wave, ready to carry you away. Who is to blame, anyway? It's quite frightening to be in the unknown and difficult to comprehend what lies ahead. It's all too much to handle, and you feel like a powerless leaf in a cyclone.

But here's the thing: the feelings you're experiencing at the moment, my friend? They are entirely typical. It's your brain's attempt to make sense of this crazy circumstance. Give yourself a break, then. Draw in a full breath. Though at times it may seem such, you are not alone in this.

You must now use your emotional intelligence to help you manage this emotional rollercoaster. It may sound sophisticated, but the main idea is to recognise your emotions and how they impact you and people around you. It's similar like learning to dance to the beat of that sentimental radio station.

The first action? Self-awareness. Pause for a moment, and consider your feelings. What effect does it have on your beliefs and behaviour? Feel free to accept those feelings without passing judgement. It's acceptable to experience vulnerability, fear, and even rage. Accepting and acknowledging them is essential if you want to begin creating a strong emotional foundation.

The next topic is self-control. It all comes down to maintaining composure when faced with hardship. I realise it's easier said than done, but there are strategies you can employ, I promise. You can learn to stabilise yourself and control your emotions by taking deep breaths, meditating, and engaging in mindfulness practises. You must figure out what works for you, whether it's journaling, going for a run, or asking for help from those you love.

But there's still more. Developing social awareness and empathy are also essential. Recall that you are not alone in navigating this storm; others are with you. Speak with those who understand you; they are aware of exactly what you are going through. Having a network of supporters provides not just affirmation but also practical advice on how to get through difficult times.

Let's now discuss hope. It like the sun making its appearance from behind ominous clouds. cling tenaciously to it, my companion. Even at the worst moments, hope is a strong force that may give you strength and encouragement. Remind yourself of the possibility of recovery and surround yourself with supportive individuals. They have faith in you as well, so you may succeed.

Remind yourself at times like this that feelings are not the enemy. They are, in actuality, markers directing you in the direction of your needs and goals. Thus, accept them. Take this rollercoaster with courage and grace, and don't be scared to do so. My friend, this is your time to grow and learn about yourself.

Emotions are ultimately the lifeblood and spirit of the Hepatitis E experience. It's a crazy journey that will put every aspect of you to the test, from hope and resilience to fear and anxiety. However, you can handle this rollercoaster by using your emotional intelligence skills, which include self-awareness, self-regulation, empathy, and social awareness. Embrace hope as if it were a lifeline, and surround yourself with like-minded people. Let's turn this adventure into a triumphant tale of self-discovery together.

The Mindful Path to Healing

Now, let's explore mindfulness and its potential benefits for managing hepatitis E. It turns out that the stress and emotional ups and downs we experience can seriously impair the function of our liver. It may exacerbate our symptoms, increase inflammation, and impede the healing process. Fortunately, research has shown that practising mindfulness can reduce stress and strengthen the immune system. For those who are coping with Hepatitis E, this is an essential tool.

What in the world is mindfulness, anyway? It all comes down to living in the present moment to the fullest and observing our thoughts, feelings, physical sensations, and the environment around us without passing judgement or being overly attached to anything. It involves merely taking a step back and observing the current situation without feeling compelled to make any adjustments or changes. Really neat, huh?

Now, let's embark on this conscious healing path. Locate a peaceful, comfortable area where you may sit or lie down without being bothered by others. Shut your eyes and inhale deeply, allowing your entire body to relax as you exhale. Feel the air entering your lungs through your nose and filling them up. And observe how each breath releases a little bit of stress.

Let's now concentrate on what's happening inside your body. Don't pass judgement on any sore spots, painful spots, or tense spots that you notice. Simply observe and accept these feelings without attempting to alter them.

Let's explore your feelings and thoughts next. Recognize the ideas that are going through your head, but try not to focus too much on them. Think of such ideas as fluffy clouds that are floating through the sky, passing by without you seeing or pondering them. Additionally, notice any feelings that surface in conjunction with those thoughts while you're doing it. Give them a sympathetic, accepting nod.

Alright, let's now turn our focus to your surroundings. Make a note of any odours, noises, or bodily sensations you encounter. Take time to truly absorb everything without assigning a label or passing judgement.

Here's the thing: it's completely normal for your thoughts to stray into the past or future. Gently bring your thoughts back to the present moment when you notice them straying from it. To help you return to reality, use your breath as an anchor.

Remind yourself to be inquisitive and present in every moment as you continue to practise mindfulness. Whatever arises, allow yourself to fully experience it without bias or attachment. Accept the present as a gift—a chance to get in touch with your inner self and discover a profound sense of contentment and well-being.

And you know what? Not only is mindfulness beneficial for mental wellness. It can also work incredibly well for your physical well-being. Numerous studies have demonstrated that practising mindfulness can strengthen your immune system, lower liver inflammation, and generally improve your mood.

According to a University of California study, those with Hepatitis C experienced less liver inflammation when they practised mindfulness-based stress reduction. Liver inflammation was lower in those who participated in the mindfulness training than in those who did not.

Another study published in the Journal of Clinical Psychology demonstrated the significant benefits of mindfulness in treating anxiety and depression. This is significant because, let's face it, Hepatitis E can seriously disrupt our emotional state and cause us to feel pessimistic about the future.

Additionally, practising mindfulness helps strengthen your immune system. How? It can, however, increase the activity of natural killer cells, which are essential in eliminating viral infections, according to study. Thus, mindfulness can assist your body in warding off that pesky Hepatitis E virus and set you on the path to recovery by strengthening your immune system.

So why not incorporate mindfulness into your daily activities? A small daily commitment of time can have a significant impact. You'll gain resilience, self-awareness, and inner tranquilly as a result of it.

And hey, try some yoga, meditation, or deep breathing techniques if you want to up your awareness game. They can provide you a well-rounded approach to managing your Hepatitis E and work in tandem with your mindfulness practise.

Recall that healing encompasses more than simply physical recovery. It's about looking after our physical and mental well-being as a whole. By adopting mindfulness and incorporating it into our daily lives, we may access this amazing ability we all possess to heal and prosper despite whatever obstacles we may encounter.

We will discuss nutrition in detail in the upcoming chapter and how it might be used to control Hepatitis E. We'll go over foods that promote liver health and lower inflammation, arming you with all the information you need to design a diet that nourishes your body and promotes healing in the event of Hepatitis E. Prepare to take control of your health and set out on a delicious path to restored energy.

Unlocking the Mind-Body Connection

Now, let's discuss the mind-body link and how it relates to the fight against hepatitis E. Understanding how our thoughts and emotions affect our physical health has advanced significantly. It's amazing to consider that our immune system, which functions as our body's barrier against diseases like hepatitis E, may be impacted by our mental health.

I mean, the mind-body connection is quite strange. The problem is that stress triggers our body's survival mode, whether it be from employment or just from our own negative thoughts and anxieties. You know, it's like fight or flight. And that sets off the release of stress chemicals like adrenaline and cortisol, which can seriously compromise our immune system.

And that's where managing Hepatitis E makes things even more crucial. While the medical aspects, such as antiviral drugs and supportive care, are undoubtedly important, we also need to consider the psychological and emotional aspects of the situation. Our immune systems can be severely compromised by stress, so we need to develop strategies to manage it.

This is the reason it's crucial to handle our health holistically. It goes beyond simply taking a few pills and going to bed. Taking a broad view, we must take into account all aspects of our lives, including our diet, physical activity, sleep patterns, stress management, and mental health.

To begin with, food. Yes, I understand that it can be tempting to bury our sorrows in an ice cream tub, but doing so won't make illnesses go away. We must eat an abundance of fruits, vegetables, whole grains, and lean meats. Additionally, certain foods like probiotics, garlic, ginger, and turmeric can help strengthen our immune systems. Thus, let's restock on those and provide our bodies with the nourishment they require to kick the ass of Hepatitis E.

Next, work out. Yes, I am aware that we don't always enjoy doing it. However, regular exercise really strengthens our immune systems, reduces stress, and generally improves our mood. The secret to this whole healing thing is finding an activity programme we genuinely enjoy, whether it's walking, working out at the gym, or doing yoga or tai chi.

Let's now discuss sleep. Yes, it's not the most glamorous subject, but it's quite significant. Our bodies begin to mend and regenerate while we sleep, and our immune systems are strengthened. However, chronic sleep deprivation weakens our immune system and increases our susceptibility to illnesses. Okay, so let's make obtaining a good night's sleep our top priority.

There's also stress management. Stress can seriously impair our mental and physical health. It's time to learn constructive coping mechanisms for that stress. Perhaps it's practising deep breathing techniques, meditation, or discovering a relaxing hobby. Let's include whatever works for us into our daily routine to manage our stress levels and prevent it from affecting our health.

Finally, but just as importantly, we need to talk about the emotional aspect of things. Receiving a diagnosis of Hepatitis E is serious business, and it's common to have feelings of fear, anxiety, or depression. Find someone to talk to, whether it's a family member, close friend, or even a professional counsellor. Don't bottle up your feelings. Hey, there are support groups out there where you can meet people experiencing similar circumstances. In this healing process, don't undervalue the importance of attending to your emotional well-being.

The basic line is that there is a real connection between our mind and body, and that connection plays a significant role in our resistance against Hepatitis E. It matters what we put into our bodies, how we move, sleep, deal with stress, and tend to our mental and emotional health. We possess the ability to strengthen our immune systems and overcome this. So let's get started.

The Healing Power of Positive Psychology

Hi and welcome to the amazing field of positive psychology! Fasten your seatbelts because we're going to discuss how adopting a positive mindset can greatly enhance your experience of controlling Hepatitis E. You're going to experience an incredible shift in your general health, my friend. With the correct attitude, you may overcome the difficulties caused by Hepatitis E with courage, resiliency, and a fierce optimism for the future.

Let's now explore the field of positive psychology science. Understanding and fostering human flourishing—happiness, wellbeing, and being the best version of oneself—is the key. Positive psychology, in contrast to traditional psychology, emphasises developing your strengths, feeling good about yourself, and being content with your life in general. My friend, our goal is to make you feel better!

First, let's discuss the influence of happy feelings. The significance those bad guys have in both your physical and mental wellbeing is significant. Positive emotions, according to research, really strengthen your immune system, lower inflammation, and help your body function as a healing machine. How then can you foster these good feelings? Easy: start a thankfulness diary. Spend a few minutes every day reflecting on all the things for which you are thankful and joyful. It might be the most beautiful sunset, a kind act from a loved one, or even the advancements you've made in controlling your Hepatitis E. By concentrating on your appreciation, you make room for more good things in your life and establish a safe haven for yourself.

Hold on, though—we're only getting started. Now let's discuss your strong points. You do indeed possess them, my friend. All of us have individual abilities and attributes that, when we allow them to flow, can improve our overall wellbeing and enable us to overcome any obstacle in our path. Using those qualities is the key to effectively managing hepatitis e. They are similar to your secret weapons—they provide you the ability to think creatively, adjust to change, and maintain a strong sense of meaning and purpose. Think back to your previous successes, moments when you felt superhuman, and the traits that got you over challenges. You may reach your greatest potential and create a strong foundation for healing and growth when you identify and celebrate your talents.

Let's now look for some direction and significance in your life. It has been demonstrated that doing this will improve your health overall. Finding meaning in life provides direction, optimism, and motivation to persevere while coping with the difficulties of controlling hepatitis E. Mindfulness is an effective tool for investigating and developing meaning. It all comes down to living in the present moment and not passing judgement on it. Spend some time focusing on your thoughts, feelings, and bodily experiences. You can find your true values and what matters to you by practising mindfulness. It's an eye-opening encounter, my friend.

Now that the scientific aspect has been discussed, let's move on to the practical. Together, we will provide you with the necessary tools and strategies to strengthen your optimistic outlook and encourage internal healing. Get set, or what? And now let's get started!

Affirmations come first. These serve as mini self-talk sessions that you do every day. Rewiring your brain to think positively about yourself and your capacity to handle Hepatitis E can be achieved by repeating affirmations. You can conquer every obstacle that comes your way because you're a strong and resilient friend. It's true, I promise!

Visualization comes next. It's similar to making a really good mental movie in which you play the lead role and visualise yourself as vibrant, healthy, and free of hepatitis E. Make use of your imagination's power to spur you on to achieve your objectives. The director of your own life is you!

Recall your thankfulness? Yes, we still have a thing for it. Every day, set aside some time to jot down three things for which you are thankful. It could be any size or shape. By engaging in this routine, you'll learn to appreciate and be content with all the good things in your life. You're the honoured guest at what resembles an appreciation party.

Finally, let us discuss self-compassion. It's not easy to live with Hepatitis E, my friend. Your body and your emotions suffer as a result. It's important to be kind, understanding, and accepting of yourself throughout those trying times. You're trying your hardest, and self-compassion promotes recovery and development. You merit it.

In summary, positive psychology is the key to effectively managing hepatitis E. Through fostering happy emotions, utilising your strengths, discovering meaning and purpose, and utilising these incredible tools and strategies, you can completely change your viewpoint and improve your general wellbeing. You may empower yourself to knock Hepatitis E in the butt with resiliency, hope, and a fresh sense of purpose by adopting these habits, my buddy. Never forget that your thoughts create your reality. Decide on optimism and allow it to lead you to the full management of Hepatitis E. You are capable!

Finding Strength in Community

Having Hepatitis E might make one feel quite alone. It is comparable to being abandoned on a desolate island, with no one nearby to sympathise with our everyday hardships. It seems like we are conversing in a foreign tongue, and our loved ones are unable to comprehend us. Finding a group of people who have experienced or are experiencing the same thing is crucial for this reason. We find a clan of kindred fighters in this group that genuinely share our dreams, concerns, and everything in between.

However, I can assure you that creating that support system is not an easy task. It requires some work and intentionality on your part. Start by making use of neighbourhood organisations and support groups that focus on Hepatitis E. You can look up suggestions on Google or get advice from your physician. These communities offer a secure space where we may share our experiences, pose inquiries, and offer support to one another. We can connect with folks who are enduring the same struggles as us by attending meetings or jumping into internet forums.

Being a part of a support system these days requires reciprocity. To receive a little, you have to give a little. Share your personal insights and guidance when you feel comfortable doing so. After all, for someone just starting out, your insights might be the light at the end of the tunnel. But remember to listen as well. Pay attentive attention to what others have to say. By doing this, we fortify the ties that bind our small town and take solace in the knowledge that we're not travelling this crazy journey alone.

The comprehension and empathy that come from having a support system is one of its greatest advantages. It is extremely difficult for others to fully understand the mental and physical toll that a chronic illness like hepatitis E puts on us. We feel like no one understands us or that we have to explain ourselves all the time. But there's no need for explanations in our tribe. Regardless of the words that leave our mouths, we see each other. We may shout from the rooftops when we overcome any setback, vent about our frustrations, and express our worst fears. We are aware that everyone listening has experienced every feeling we are, and that is very remarkable.

But there's still more! Not everything about our little village is sentimental. It has some useful advice under its sleeve as well. Our fellow combatants are knowledgeable. They have been in the trenches, trying out various coping strategies, therapeutic approaches, and adjustments to their way of life. They have some manoeuvres up their sleeves that we may not have even considered. Naturally, we must keep in mind that a warrior's strategy may differ from another's. Thus, consult your physician before attempting anything new. However, having this community as our own source of learning... It is quite lovely.

Let's now discuss those times when it seems like the entire world is resting on our shoulders. Sometimes a chronic condition can truly take the wind out of our sails. Having a support system in place during difficult times is even more crucial. We discover courage and strength we never knew we had when we confide in people who genuinely get us. The neighbourhood comes together for us, offering words of support and sharing personal accounts of their own resiliency. They serve as a reminder that, despite any challenges we may face, we are able to pick ourselves up and carry on.

What more do you know? The community isn't limited to its presence during difficult times. When the good times come, they're by our sides as well. The community joins us in celebrating successes when we reach new heights of wellbeing or nail a treatment plan for Hepatitis E. They understand the enormity of these accomplishments and the blood, sweat, and tears that were shed to get there. That mutual happiness gives us a boost and strengthens our self-belief. It's definitely a reminder that we have a large group of individuals rooting for us and ready to support us.

In summary, overcoming Hepatitis E requires seeking support in a community. Building that support system allows you to access knowledge, compassion, and helpful advice from those who have been there before. Their combined knowledge provides us with the fortitude and resources we need to handle the highs and lows of this crazy adventure. We ensure we have all the support we need to overcome this Hepatitis E struggle by coming together and finding comfort, inspiration, and hope.

Building a Support Network

Finding Your Tribe

Having Hepatitis E might make you feel as though you are stranded on a remote island. The general public frequently has misconceptions about this illness, which makes it difficult for them to fully appreciate the effects it has on our lives. Even those closest to us, despite their best efforts, find it difficult to completely comprehend the mental and physical toll it takes on us. Finding a tribe, or a group of individuals who truly get it and are deeply aware of what it means to have Hepatitis E, is crucial for this reason.

Upon discovering that I had Hepatitis E, I felt as though my entire world had collapsed. I felt like I was on my own because none of my close friends or relatives had experienced this. I felt disoriented, perplexed, and overpowered. But then, as fate would have it, I happened into an internet support group for Hepatitis E sufferers. And that really did change everything, I swear to you.

For me, it was a turning point to join the organisation. All of a sudden, I found myself surrounded by a group of warriors who were cognizant of both the mental and physical rollercoaster I was experiencing. When I most needed it, these people—my tribe—gave me courage and hope. And I want to show you how transforming it may be to find your tribe in this section.

First of all, it's vital to identify people who can genuinely relate to you and provide emotional support. The fear, anxiety, and depressing times that come with having Hepatitis E can be quite taxing. However, belonging to a tribe entails being around by others who experience the same emotional ups and downs. They experience all of it as well, including periods of hopelessness, worry, and terror. And let me tell you, knowing that you're not travelling alone on this road is tremendously comforting.

It seemed like a weight had been taken off my shoulders when I first discovered my tribe. They applauded my little wins, understood my fears, and spoke the same language as me. Their inspirational tales of tenacity offered me hope and served as a reminder that I was strong enough to carry on. The best thing, though? I could express my own feelings without worrying about being rejected or judged. I could be vulnerable there since it was a secure place.

But discovering your tribe has benefits beyond just providing emotional support. Making connections with people who have gone through similar things to you can lead to a wealth of useful advice and techniques. Let's face it: having Hepatitis E has its own unique set of difficulties. And getting around them often seems like attempting to untangle an endless skein of thread. However, you'll discover a plethora of communal knowledge that can genuinely transform lives inside your tribe.

I discovered a plethora of useful answers in my tribe. My tribe was a wealth of information, covering everything from food adjustments to lifestyle adjustments, stress reduction methods to substitutes for self-care. The extent to which it enhanced my general well-being is beyond words. Together, with the support of our distinct viewpoints and life experiences, we discovered methods that helped lessen flare-ups, lessen symptoms, and enhance our quality of life. It was similar to finding a hidden playbook that altered the course of events.

The sensation of belonging that comes with discovering your tribe, though, is its greatest advantage. Having Hepatitis E might make you feel alienated and as though you're fighting a war that few people truly comprehend. You are not alone, though, in your tribe. People who appreciate and comprehend you for who you are are all around you. I will never forget the surge of warmth and welcome I experienced when I walked into my first Hepatitis E support group meeting. We told our tales, laughed, and we grieved together without needing to rationalise or explain anything. It was a really amazing occasion.

It was a mental and emotional game-changer to find my tribe. Some of the closest friends I have are the ones I made in this group. Together, we have encouraged and supported one another during this journey's highs and lows. Our unshakable friendship was created by our common experiences and awareness of the difficulties we confront. I now possess resilience, strength, and a renewed sense of self-worth thanks to my community.

Therefore, I implore anyone beginning their adventure with Hepatitis E to locate their tribe. Finding your tribe can be achieved in a variety of ways, such as through local meet-ups, online support groups, or social media connections with people who have gone through similar situations. You'll discover useful tips, emotional support, and—above all—a feeling of community. You'll come to realise a strength you never knew you had. I want you to realise the tremendous importance of discovering your tribe in this section. It completes your strategy for overcoming hepatitis E by giving you the support and confidence you require at every turn.

Support Groups: A Lifeline

As a physician and health and wellness coach, I have to admit that I've witnessed some pretty incredible things in my work. And the amazing power of support groups is one of those things. It truly seems like magic is occurring before my very eyes. I want to take you on a tour today to learn about the various support groups that are accessible for people with hepatitis E. You won't want to miss this journey, I can assure you of that.

First up, the tried-and-true in-person support groups. Imagine that a room full of people are gathering to discuss their experiences, struggles, and victories. Everyone can express themselves freely there without fear of being judged. I still recall going to this one support group meeting with my patient, Robin.

As soon as we entered the room, the atmosphere was one of warmth and companionship. A few months prior, Robin, a thirty-something lady, had received her Hepatitis E diagnosis. She was having a lot of difficulty accepting it. But what's the deal? This support system turned into her lifesaver. She felt comfortable discussing her worries, her frustrations, and her hopes there. And believe me when I say that that room was full of people from all different backgrounds, each with a distinct tale to tell.

The way these people interacted and comforted one another most amazed me. There was this guy named Mike who had been struggling with Hepatitis E for more than ten years until Robin opened up about how it was harming her career. He had some wisdom to impart, I must say. He covered workplace navigation, telling your supervisor and coworkers about your condition, and advocating for adjustments. He resembled a living, breathing encyclopaedia of all things related to hepatitis E.

However, they didn't just share useful tips, you know? It also provided emotional support. Emma was a woman who spoke about how having Hepatitis E made her anxious and depressed. And believe me when I say that this atmosphere of understanding and empathy was fostered by that vulnerability. People reassured one another that it's perfectly acceptable to seek professional assistance, such as therapy and counselling, discussed their own experiences, and offered coping mechanisms to one another.

Support groups now serve more purposes than merely sharing and consoling. They also aim to provide people with useful materials. Similar to this occasion, when a local hepatitis association official stopped over to discuss the most recent developments in Hepatitis E treatment. It felt as invigorating as a rush of wind. The members experienced empowerment and even hope. They came to see that others were trying to improve their lives and that they weren't the only ones on this trip.

But there's still more! Not to be overlooked are the internet support groups. People who have Hepatitis E can communicate with others who are going through similar things, wherever in the world, because of the internet. These online groups provide constant dialogue, resource sharing, and emotional support; they're like a lifeline.

I have personal experience with the life-changing power of internet support groups. Consider Sarah as an example. She resided in a distant location with little access to medical treatment and specialist support networks. But she was able to connect with a large network of others who were aware of her troubles by joining an online Hepatitis E support group. They offered her guidance on coping mechanisms, complementary therapies, and self-care. She gained the confidence and sense of empowerment from that online group to successfully manage her Hepatitis E journey.

For those with Hepatitis E, support groups—whether they be in-person or virtual—are like a lifeline. They establish this secure environment where people can tell their stories without fear of rejection or shame. However, they provide more than just information exchange; they also provide tools, resources, and the most recent findings and developments in medicine. However, their perseverance, sense of belonging, and sense of hope are what truly set them apart.

It can truly change your life to realise that you're not alone and that there are people out there who understand your challenges. No matter how bad things become, there's always hope for a better tomorrow thanks to the experiences and tales shared in these support groups. And believe me when I say that you don't want to overlook the importance of support groups.

We'll delve into the realm of self-care and examine several methods and approaches to effectively manage Hepatitis E in the upcoming chapter. So check back soon for a whole manual on holistic self-care for managing hepatitis E. I promise, it will be fantastic.

The Power of Online Communities

Allow me to share with you the amazing benefits that online communities offer to those living with Hepatitis E. I can attest to the loneliness and isolation that often accompany a chronic illness. Friends and relatives may not always understand the difficulties and obstacles we experience on a daily basis due to Hepatitis E. However, virtual societies? They provide a saviour. They provide us with a forum for interacting with people who share our experiences and have travelled a similar path. We take comfort in the knowledge that we're not fighting this battle alone and a sense of belonging from those virtual relationships.

And these virtual groups offer us more than simply consolation. They are veritable gold mines of information. As you can see, people in the community talk about their experiences, coping techniques, and approaches to treatment. It's comparable to a mine of potentially game-changing revelations. Particularly for people who are having trouble managing their illness or have just received a diagnosis. We can ask questions, look for assistance, and gain knowledge from the experiences of others who have faced similar challenges by participating in online forums. That gives you power, my friend. It provides us with the knowledge and resources we need to manage our Hepatitis E journey.

That's not all, though. These virtual communities serve as venues for awareness-raising and education as well. We keep up with the most recent developments and innovations in the industry. Novel therapeutic approaches, clinical studies, preemptive actions... Everything is shared inside these virtual borders. By educating others, we give ourselves and others more power. Additionally, we are vital in dispelling the stigma associated with Hepatitis E and increasing public knowledge of the disease. And what's this? Increased awareness can result in better treatment outcomes, early detection, and a society where people are not ashamed of their condition.

Allow me to illustrate with an actual case. Introducing Sarah. The young lady received a diagnosis of Hepatitis E. Just think of how bewildered and overwhelmed she must have felt. But she refused to let it get to her. Nope, she resorted to social media groups and online forums. She discovered people who had been dealing with Hepatitis E for years in those online groups. And they greeted Sarah with wide arms, my buddy. She was really comforted and guided by their sharing of their experiences and tales. She gained knowledge on food modifications, lifestyle changes, and coping mechanisms that have been successful for other people. Equipped with this assistance and understanding, she crafted a customised self-care regimen that enhanced her standard of living. That is powerful stuff, isn't it?

However, do you know what's even more potent? the opposite. Introducing John. Although he made a different decision, he received the same diagnosis as Sarah. John made the decision to withdraw, be solitary, and refrain from contacting internet support groups. Believe me when I say that it wasn't easy for him. He was drowned in a sea of information overload, feeling bewildered and alone. His experience with Hepatitis E turned into a never-ending cycle of frustration and uncertainty without the support of online forums.

The divergent experiences of John and Sarah provide powerful tales of the transforming power of online forums for the Hepatitis E community. Those like Sarah who sign up for these online support groups discover a group of people who relate to and affirm their experiences. However, it doesn't end there. These networks also provide us with information and tools, enabling us to create efficient plans for managing our illness. And what else, you know? They give us a stage on which to speak up for one another and ourselves. We produce a voice that is unavoidable.

I therefore cannot emphasise enough how crucial internet groups are to the Hepatitis E community, my buddy. They provide us with a network of support, the resources we require to manage our illness, and a voice to advocate for what is rightfully ours. Look, don't wait to get help if you or someone you know has Hepatitis E. Explore these virtual communities. By working together, we can create a community that is brave, empowered, and supportive. We can defeat hepatitis E together.

Nurturing Personal Relationships

Living with Hepatitis E can make you feel as though you're alone and in the dark. It can be debilitating, lonely, and even frightening at times. You distance yourself from the people that matter to you because you don't want to bother them with your problems. This causes an invisible wall to form between you and them. But hear me out, friend: you can never undervalue the ability of close friendships to keep you afloat when you feel like you're going under.

Being upfront with your loved ones is crucial when you have Hepatitis E. Tell them your diagnosis and open your world to them. Assist them in comprehending the physical and mental suffering you're experiencing. Spread it all out on the table, and see how they come together to support you without reservation.

The problem is that they might not understand it at first. Not exactly a conversation starter at the dinner table, hepatitis E. Thus, spend some time educating them. Provide articles, resources, or anything else that will aid in their understanding of your disease. By providing them with information, you're providing them with the means by which they can actually understand what you're up against.

Remember to establish boundaries as well. Living with Hepatitis E necessitates some lifestyle alterations, which you must be sure to share with your loved ones. Tell them when you need to sleep, when you need help, and when you need a bit more tolerance. You're taking charge of your health and avoiding undue stress on yourself by establishing these boundaries.

But keep in mind that partnerships are two-way. It goes beyond simply meeting your needs. It's possible that your loved ones will need to lower their expectations or look for outside assistance. It involves making concessions and striking a balance between your well-being and theirs. Thus, maintain open channels of communication and come up with ideas that satisfy all parties.

Additionally, don't be afraid to call out to others outside of your immediate circle for assistance if you need it. Enroll in a support group or look for Hepatitis E-specific counselling options. These safe spaces can be your lifeline—people who can offer you helpful advice and coping mechanisms in addition to understanding what you're going through. You'll create a network of people who will encourage you when things become hard and help you when you need it most.

Finally, never undervalue the influence of sharing your personal stories. You're not only enhancing your relationship with your loved ones by talking about your experience with Hepatitis E, but you're also reducing the stigma associated with this illness. People must hear your narrative and witness personally your tenacity and fortitude. It might possibly alter their viewpoint, which would then alter how society perceives hepatitis E.

Thus, my friend, treasure those close bonds. Despite their difficulties, they are well worth the effort. You are not defined by hepatitis E, and it most definitely does not define your social skills. You'll find the fortitude and resiliency you need to get through this trip by fostering the relationships with the people you love and who want to be there for you. You can do this.

Self-Care: A Foundation of Support

I've been practising self-care for a while now, and I can honestly say that it has changed my life. Taking deliberate steps to look after your physical, emotional, mental, and spiritual needs is the essence of self-care. It's an absolute necessity—especially if you have a condition like hepatitis E—rather than a flashy luxury. Setting self-care as a top priority may, I promise, change your life. It's like creating a solid support system you can rely on in difficult times.

Mindfulness is an essential component of self-care. It all comes down to being totally present in the here and now, detached from judgement or attachment. And believe me when I say that practising mindfulness on a regular basis may completely transform your life. It improves your mental health, eases tension and anxiety, and lets you unwind. Mindfulness practises such as deep breathing, eating with awareness, and meditation can help you if you're fighting Hepatitis E. You can manage all the mental and physical turbulence this illness throws at you by remaining in the now and maintaining your composure.

Now, as physical health is equally vital, let's discuss it. Exercise on a regular basis not only improves your physical health but also has a profound effect on your mental and emotional wellness. Stress is eliminated and joyful endorphins are released. It's important to speak with your healthcare providers and develop an exercise regimen that suits your needs if you have Hepatitis E. Whatever it is that makes you happy and contributes to your overall health—a stroll, some yoga, or low-impact exercise—you're doing great.

Hey, there's another major participant in the self-care game: nutrition. It's essential to have a balanced diet that promotes liver health and promotes recovery. Speak with your medical providers to receive a customised diet plan that meets your requirements. Include foods that nourish your liver, such as fruits high in antioxidants, leafy greens, and healthy fats. And please, for the love of everything that is good, avoid processed meals and alcohol, as they will put stress on your liver. Your body will appreciate you if you give it what it needs.

What else is important in self-care, do you know? methods for relaxation. It's essential to engage in activities that allow you to decompress, reduce tension, and simply relax. Deep breathing exercises, taking warm baths, engaging in creative or artistic endeavours, or simply spending time in nature are all like a miraculous remedy for all the problems that Hepatitis E might hurl at you. I can assure you that if you make relaxation a regular part of your life, you'll experience reduced stress, improved emotional health, and a network of supportive people.

However, self-care is a freaking journey rather than merely a collection of techniques. Permit me to share Sarah's storey with you. When Sarah, a young lady, was initially diagnosed with hepatitis E, she was terrified and unsure of what lay ahead. She then made the decision to put self-care first, and let me tell you, that completely transformed her life. She began to exercise gently, practise mindfulness, and fuel her body with healthy foods. And what's this? Painting gave her comfort, something she hadn't done in a long time. Sarah's support system expanded as well, and she began to feel stronger and more in control. Sarah encouraged those with Hepatitis E to emphasise self-care and discover their own road to wellness by sharing her storey.

You see, developing your resilience and fortifying your support system are the cornerstones of self-care. Exercise, healthy eating, mindfulness, and relaxation techniques are just a few of the habits that can significantly improve your mental and physical health. People living with Hepatitis E can discover inspiration and direction to confront their path with strength and confidence through personal tales and the power of self-care. Folks, take note: self-care is an absolute requirement and should not be disregarded. Accept it and observe how you overcome obstacles in your path.

Navigating Stigma and Discrimination

The shame and discrimination associated with having Hepatitis E cast a pall over their lives. Although there has been progress in medicine, this illness affects not only one's bodily health but also one's mental and emotional stability. The lack of knowledge regarding Hepatitis E in many communities is frustrating. Ignorance gives rise to inaccurate information and damaging stereotypes that exacerbate the situation. People become ashamed, alone, and feel alienated as a result of it.

But what's the deal? Personal narrative is one way that can shine a bright light through that barrier. Hepatitis E patients personalise the illness and confront preconceived notions when they share details about their experiences. They may demonstrate to the world via their stories the struggles they face, the challenges they overcome, and their inner strength. These tales serve as a reminder to everybody that hepatitis E does not define its carriers. They are complex people deserving of consideration and compassion.

Emily is one person who truly made an impression on me. At the ripe old age of 25, she was diagnosed with Hepatitis E while she was just beginning her legal career. It seemed as though everything had abruptly turned upside down. She first concealed it out of fear that her clients and coworkers would reject her. But as the symptoms began to seriously damage her health, she came to the realisation that she had to face reality head-on.

Fearless warrior that she is, Emily made the decision to face that stigma head-on. She started a blog where she shared the good, bad, and ugly of her journey. And what's this? It was an amazing response. Individuals emerged from the shadows to provide their support and share their personal accounts of coping with long-term illness. Emily came to see that speaking up not only brought her peace but also fostered empathy and understanding among others.

Emily's storey is a prime illustration of the persuasiveness of personal storytelling. People like her can break down social barriers that encourage discrimination and educate others about the difficulties they confront by sharing their stories. Their experiences develop empathy and build an inclusive society for all people, regardless of their medical issues.

Additionally, the general public needs to be made aware about hepatitis E. People have this bizarre assumption that irresponsible behaviour or poor cleanliness are the only causes. These untrue notions simply serve to propagate guilt and blame, which breed prejudice. We need to provide people with correct information on the causes, transmission, and treatment of hepatitis E if we want to change the narrative.

It is my responsibility as a medical professional and a health and wellness coach to provide my patients with the resources they need to deal with discrimination and stigma. Giving kids the confidence to defend others as well as themselves is one effective tool. Hepatitis E patients can find strength in their own tales, just as Emily did when she used her blog to discover her voice.

But narrative nonfiction is not the only thing here. We also need to disseminate knowledge. Workshops, instructional materials, and community outreach can help us achieve that. Through providing precise facts, we can dispel the falsehoods and misunderstandings that give rise to stigma. Armed with that information, people may boldly confront prejudice, enlighten others, and create an inclusive society.

We also need to establish support networks. People with Hepatitis E need safe places to talk about their experiences, find solace, and discuss coping mechanisms. These networks provide a lifeline, supporting the development of resilience against discrimination and assisting in the fight against loneliness.

In order to successfully navigate the tangle that is stigma and discrimination, counselling and psychological help are also critical. It's a fact that having a chronic illness has an impact on our mental and emotional health. Mental health specialists can assist people in overcoming the emotional effects of stigma, improving their self-esteem, and coping. Through counselling, people can gain the skills necessary to dispel stigma, educate others, and open doors to acceptance and understanding.

Through therapy, education, support groups, and personal accounts, individuals with Hepatitis E can effectively negotiate the complex terrain of stigma and discrimination. By speaking up, individuals are promoting social change in addition to standing up for themselves. My goal as a physician and health and wellness coach is to empower people and accompany them on their path to knowledge, acceptance, and a day when prejudice and stigma will no longer control us.

Lifestyle Modifications

The Battle Against the Bottle

Chapter 7: The Battle Against the Bottle

Subchapter: Conquering Alcohol Addiction for Better Liver Health

Introduction:

Now, for the catch. Alcoholism is a serious illness. Many of us fight this war in private, saying we're just having fun or attempting to take our sorrow away. However, I assure you that it is not worthwhile. Our bodies suffer greatly from this addiction, particularly our livers. I can attest that the damage is real since I have personally witnessed it. That's the reason I'm here, as a doctor and a health and wellness coach, to share my experience with you, offer guidance, and support you in making important positive changes in your life.

My Personal Journey:

To begin with, I would like to clarify that I did not become an alcoholic overnight. It started off simply enough, as a way to enjoy the good times or relax after a long day. But over time, it turned became my go-to. I became dependent on it as a coping mechanism for tension and worry, and before I knew it, my liver was suffering greatly. My eyes went yellow, my stomach ached, and I became constantly tired—all classic symptoms of liver disease.

I was awakened by that. I could not deny that I was the reason for my own decline in health. I decided to change my life as a result. It wasn't easy, but I went to support groups, asked friends and family for guidance, and sought assistance from addiction counsellors. I was ultimately able to overcome my addiction with perseverance and drive.

The Link between Alcohol and Hepatitis E:

Now for the terrifying part, guys. Hepatitis E and alcohol go hand in hand, but not in a positive way. You see, consuming alcohol by itself might damage your liver, but when Hepatitis E is involved, things get worse. This terrible virus targets your liver directly, causing inflammation that results in the development of Hepatitis E. And you know what? Studies reveal that drinking too much alcohol increases your risk of contracting Hepatitis E and its very unpleasant symptoms.

Because alcohol depletes your immune system, Hepatitis E can spread more easily. Furthermore, it interferes with your body's capacity to absorb nutrients that are essential for your liver to function correctly. It's akin to a double whammy: alcohol weakens your liver and interferes with your immune system, which makes it ideal for that nasty virus to spread.

Practical Tips and Strategies:

Alright, enough of the eerie details. Let's discuss how to defeat this obstacle. Alcohol addiction recovery calls for a variety of approaches, but I'm here to provide you some doable advice that will truly help. So pay attention:

1. Seek Professional Help: See, I understand. Addiction is serious business, and we occasionally require expert assistance to overcome it. Thus, get in touch with those addiction counsellors or sign up for support groups so you may receive the direction and assistance you require.

2. Build a Supportive Network: My friend, you cannot handle this by yourself. Be in the company of those who can sympathise with you and lend a supporting hand. It might be your friends, family, or even internet groups. Just be sure you have a support system in place to help you when you need it.

3. Identify Triggers and Create Alternatives: You know those moments or feelings that make you want to sip alcohol? Yes, that's where we've all been. The challenge is to look for healthier substitutes. It could be taking up a new activity, exercising, or

practising meditation. Don't reach for the bottle; instead, do whatever helps you relax and de-stress.

4. Practice Self-Care Techniques: It's crucial that you look after yourself. Establish a schedule that promotes your mental, emotional, and physical well. Maintain a journal, engage in mindfulness exercises, get adequate sleep, and make sure you're feeding your body healthful foods. It all comes down to taking care of oneself.

5. Set Realistic Goals: I want you to pay close attention now. Try not to complete it all at once. Start off small and reduce your alcohol consumption over time. Establish attainable objectives and acknowledge each small victory as you proceed. I promise you that every step you take to cut less on alcohol is good for your liver.

6. Develop Coping Strategies: It's a hard life, and obstacles are inevitable. So, acquire good coping mechanisms for stress and difficulties. Perhaps you could attempt counselling or alternative therapies like massage or acupuncture. Perhaps it simply comes down to enjoying the things that bring you joy. Choose your coping strategy and stay with it, whatever that may be.

Conclusion:

The truth is that overcoming an alcohol addiction is a difficult but worthwhile path. It will not only help your liver, but it will also enable you to take back your general health. Knowing the risky link between alcohol and Hepatitis E equips you with the information you need to make wise decisions for the health of your liver. And by putting these useful advice and techniques into practice—like getting expert assistance, creating a network of allies, and creating coping mechanisms—you're positioning yourself for success. Recall that every step you take to cut back on alcohol is a step toward a healthier liver, and that it is never too late to begin this recovery road.

Continue reading in Chapter 8: Nourishing the Liver: A Holistic Approach to Diet and Lifestyle Modifications.

The Hidden Dangers of Alcohol

You know, the liver functions inside our bodies like this amazing superhero. It performs all these important tasks, including metabolism, detoxification, and even the synthesis of some essential chemicals. But yeah, that liver of ours gets beat up when we start beating back the alcohol like it's no big deal. Things can start to go very wrong when it becomes very agitated and heated.

This inflammation that develops in the liver when we drink far too much alcohol is known as alcoholic hepatitis. It can range from mild discomfort to outright anarchy, and it can get very savage at times. And let me tell you, these are not to be taken lightly symptoms: fever, jaundice, and stomach ache are all present. But that alcoholic hepatitis can get worse if we just let it ride. At that point, cirrhosis comes into play.

My friend, cirrhosis is the condition in which scar tissue begins to replace your healthy liver cells. Yes, scar tissue—you heard me right. That material acts as a bully, pushing out the beneficial elements and interfering with your liver's ability to function. It's also not a transient problem. You will always have cirrhosis, and it is a one-way path. Indeed, if you believed that drinking alcohol was merely a small annoyance for those who had Hepatitis E, you should reconsider. A small amount of it can hasten the progression of cirrhosis in a person who has previously been afflicted with hepatitis E.

I recall one of my patients, Mr. Thompson, who had Hepatitis E but was unable to stop drinking alcohol despite my warnings. The man simply continued to chug. And what took place? His liver plummeted, plunging straight into cirrhosis. Unfortunately, Mr. Thompson's experience is not unique; I have witnessed several Hepatitis E patients fight this same battle and be unable to kick alcohol out of their lives.

Tell me about someone, though, who did saw the light and decided to make a change. Sarah was a young, gregarious person who enjoyed going out and having a few drinks with her pals. But she made a decision, guy, when she discovered she had Hepatitis E. She stopped drinking altogether, as if it never happened.

Observe what transpired. In just a few months, Sarah had completely changed. Fresh as ever, her liver was back in action. Her energy levels shot through the roof, and those pesky Hepatitis E symptoms? Man, they disappeared. It resembled magic. I only needed to look at Sarah's change to be convinced that the best course of action for someone with Hepatitis E was to refuse alcohol.

And believe me when I say that science is on our side. Research has repeatedly demonstrated that drinking alcohol and having Hepatitis E can be extremely harmful. If you continue to use alcohol while having Hepatitis E, your chances of developing cirrhosis are significantly increased. Additionally, alcohol has a tendency of compromising our immune systems, making it more difficult for us to fight against the hepatitis virus and taxing our liver further.

So, people, you need to realise how crucial it is to put alcohol on the back burner if you have Hepatitis E. It's all about allowing your liver to recuperate and keeping things from going out of control. In my field, I usually emphasise the need of addressing Hepatitis E with a comprehensive strategy. It's not only about what you consume in your mouth; it's also about altering your way of life, coming up with fresh coping mechanisms, and yes, seeking out psychological support.

The good news is that many people with Hepatitis E have experienced significant improvements in their liver health by reducing their alcohol consumption. It all comes down to coming up with fresh strategies for handling stress and acknowledging small victories along the road. Well, it's not always simple, but managing your health in that way can have a profound impact on your general wellbeing.

In conclusion, folks, pay attention. Hepatitis E and alcohol don't mix, just like oil and water. Your liver can suffer greatly from alcohol consumption, from inflammation to cirrhosis. I've told you about a few of my patients' experiences and presented some credible data to emphasise how important it is to limit alcohol use if you want to manage Hepatitis E. Thus, take command, my friend, and show your liver the respect and affection it so richly deserves. Your life will appreciate it, I promise.

Clearing the Smoke

In my work as a physician and wellness advocate, I have witnessed some fairly depressing things. Smoking's terrible effects on liver health are one item that truly bothers me. Similar to how other, more evident concerns like lung cancer and heart disease tend to overwhelm this silent danger, it is frequently disregarded. It's no laughing matter, though, as smoking and liver conditions such as Hepatitis E are closely related.

Imagine the following: A cigarette lights up, you take a drag, and suddenly these feel-good, happy-making chemicals rush your brain. That's correct—nicotine deceives your brain into experiencing increasing cravings like a cunning little demon. It's quite difficult to stop smoking because of this. Here's the thing, though: most smokers are unaware of the extent of the harm they are causing to their liver.

A tonne of harmful substances that invade our bodies are present in those cigarettes. Consider the gas carbon monoxide. The ability of our red blood cells to transmit oxygen is disrupted when this tiny pest adheres to them. Whoa, what now? For optimal function, our liver cells require that oxygen. Hence, smoking basically depletes our liver of oxygen and gradually tampers with its equilibrium. There is also acrolein, a poisonous substance that damages our liver and irritates our respiratory system. These smokes seem like tiny, dangerous packages that are just ready to wreak havoc on our livers.

It's at this point when things truly start to go south. Smoking and hepatitis e are a dangerous combination that can only end badly. An unpleasant virus that spreads through tainted food or water is the source of the hepatitis E infection. Your initial symptoms could be mild exhaustion, appetite loss, or nausea. However, the virus has the potential to cause havoc on your liver if you smoke and do not treat it appropriately. Hepatic failure is a serious issue that requires careful consideration, my buddy.

With a brief anecdote, allow me to explain. Adam was a patient of mine in the past. Who knew that the poor guy had been diagnosed with Hepatitis E? Chain smoking was his habit. Without even recognising that his daily pack of cigarettes was damaging his liver, he continued to smoke. Initially, there was no need for concern as his Hepatitis E was quite minor. But because of his smoking habit, things quickly got out of hand. His liver was simply overtaken by the virus and the harmful substances from the cigarettes. Poor Adam, he had just given up smoking, and now all he had to do was regret it. It was a one-way ticket to liver failure.

It may seem unattainable to give up smoking, but I assure you that it is feasible. That inner drive is something you must discover. Consider your reasons for wanting to give up. Do you want to take back control of your life, save your loved ones, or improve your health? To overcome those insane cravings, my buddy, discover the fire within you.

However, you are not required to work alone. Assemble a small support network around yourself. They're all there to support you during the hard times: friends, family, and support groups. Remember to give yourself a deadline to stop. Formalize it. Put an end to your cigarette habit and begin a new journey.

Not to mention that well-known quit strategy. Customize it to meet your needs and make it your own. Try some healthy cigarette substitutes, start an exercise regimen, or engage in mindfulness techniques to find inner tranquilly. Please don't hesitate to contact an expert if you require any additional assistance. It's critical to confront our individual triggers head-on because we are all different.

Friends, hold yourself responsible. Make sure you monitor your advancement and acknowledge each small victory as you go. Are you smoke-free for a week now? What an incredible! It's been a month now. Yes, absolutely! Your determination to live a better lifestyle is strengthened by every step you take in lieu of smoking cigarettes.

Do not forget to look after yourself. Encounter happiness in the small things that give you a sense of life. Activities you enjoy, whether it be yoga, meditation, or hobbies. You can finally give up smoking if you take care of your mental and emotional health.

It's time for me to be honest. Those cravings will occasionally strike hard. Especially when life becomes hectic, they have the ability to surprise you and ambush you. For them, though, you must be prepared. Inhale deeply, rely on your support system, and employ constructive coping techniques. This is yours.

We can stop smoking and give our livers a better chance if we work together. Every step you take to stop smoking is a step toward regaining the health of your liver and leading a purposeful life. So, my friend, let's clarify the air. Let's break free from the shackles of smoking by arming ourselves with information and resources. Free from the chains of smoking, let's restore the health of our livers and lead the greatest lives possible. Let us proceed.

Breaking Free From the Smoking Trap

I was full of life, young, and knowledgeable about illnesses, their causes, and their remedies. I believed I was immune to the very diseases I researched, making me untouchable. However, I had no idea that the things I was doing were taking me down a dangerous path. It all began quite simply, with the occasional cigarette during get-togethers. I saw it as a means of blending in with the group. However, one cigarette quickly became two, then three, and before I knew it, I was addicted.

I was first unaware of the damage smoking was doing to my health. I told myself that the episodes of coughing and dyspnea were only minor inconveniences. But I knew deep down that smoking was killing me, slowly but certainly. It was destroying my physical health in addition to my mental health.

Then I was struck down hard by fate. One day, while going through a patient's medical files, I came across a case of chronic smoking-related liver illness. It was a revelation that struck me like a brick. The fact that I would also have a damaged liver if I persisted on this dangerous path was unavoidable. I had seen the terrible consequences of liver disease firsthand, and I didn't want that for my own life.

The process of giving up smoking then started. It was a hard battle upward. The physical dependence on nicotine was only the beginning. The hardest chains to break turned out to be the psychological ones. Smoking had evolved from a habit to my crutch, a coping mechanism for boredom, tension, and worry. I have to reprogram my brain to handle these feelings in a healthier way.

I turned to my network of support for comfort. I talked to my friends, coworkers, and family about my troubles. Their support and empathy turned into my lifeline. They inspired me to keep going even on the worst of days by serving as a reminder of my own strength.

Armed with useful resources and strategies, I took on the cravings and symptoms of withdrawal head-on. When the temptation to smoke struck, deep breathing exercises became my saving grace. I would visualise all the poisons leaving my body as I closed my eyes, took a deep breath, and slowly exhaled. This small gesture gave me back control over my emotions and breathing.

I distracted my hands and head with other things to take my mind off desires. Everywhere I went, I had a stress ball with me, and whenever temptation struck, I would squeeze it. And I found comfort in creative endeavours like writing and painting. By expressing my feelings via art, I was able to let go of my anxiety and achieve peace of mind.

However, visualising proved to be one of my most effective tools in my recuperation. I would close my eyes and visualise living a life devoid of tobacco. I could picture myself having a lively liver, strong lungs, and a life full of vigour and energy. I was able to stay focused on my objectives because I could see the amazing benefits that awaited me after I overcome my addiction.

I was unable to ignore the improvements in my health as the days grew into weeks and the weeks into months. Eventually, my cough went away and I was able to breathe deeply again without experiencing any pain. I was no longer smelling like smoke, and the residual tobacco smell had left my clothes and hair. Most crucially, though, my liver function improved. It was starting to mend because the toxins that had formerly overtaken it were starting to recede.

Leaving the smoking trap was a metamorphosis for my resiliency and sense of self-worth in addition to my physical wellbeing. I came to realise that I had the ability to transform my life and overcome every challenge that stood in my way. This increased self-assurance stoked my desire to assist others in achieving the same.

I hope to motivate and inspire people to escape the smoking trap by sharing my own path. I want people to know that they are capable of taking back control of their health and liver function and that they have the strength and resources to do it. Anyone can start their own journey to a smoke-free life by using doable strategies, techniques, and in-depth self-reflection.

In summary, breaking free from the addiction to smoking is a difficult but worthwhile journey. Anyone may break free from the psychological and physical bonds of addiction by looking for help, using useful skills and strategies, and picturing a better future. Living a smoke-free life has several advantages beyond improved liver function. It's a chance to take back control, embrace self-determination, and lead a full, vibrant life. So, now is the day to take that courageous first step and start your own road toward emancipation.

Fueling Your Body With Nutrition

Treatment for Hepatitis E is not the only thing that is needed. Giving your body the proper nourishment to fight back is the key. And you know what? In this tale, the liver takes on a heroic role. It's the ultimate detoxifier, and the secret to treating Hepatitis E is keeping your liver healthy. Now let's explore the world of nutrition and treat your liver with the respect it so richly merits.

The liver is a tiny, ravenous organ that requires a wide variety of nutrients in order to function properly. We are discussing healthy fats, vitamins, minerals, and antioxidants. Imagine them as the Avengers, prepared to kick some free radicals and save your liver. Not only will these nutrients strengthen your liver, but they will also boost your immunity and hasten your recuperation when added to your meals.

Antioxidants function similarly to the shield that protects your liver from free radical damage. Why is it important to worry about free radicals? These little miscreants have the potential to induce oxidative stress, which can harm the liver and cause inflammation. Not good. Antioxidants, however, can counteract these free radicals and protect your liver, so don't worry. So where are these potent antioxidants found? You only need to look at fruits, vegetables, nuts, and seeds. Antioxidants resemble the Justice League of superheroes.

Berries, citrus fruits, and grapes are among the fruits that are rich in vitamin C and flavonoids, which are potent antioxidants that reduce inflammation and maintain the health of your liver. Imagine a bowl full of mixed berries that are so vibrant and flavorful they will make your liver happy.

Not to mention our green leafy heroes, broccoli, kale, and spinach. These nasty boys are loaded with nutrients like zinc and selenium along with vitamins A, C, and E. They give your liver the vigour it needs to detox and remain healthy, much like the Hulk.

Naturally, we also can't ignore our sleazy and goofy sidekicks. Rich in omega-3 fatty acids and other good fats, walnuts, almonds, and chia seeds are excellent sources of antioxidants. These men improve the functionality of your liver and reduce inflammation, kind of like Robin to Batman. For that extra, amazing boost, don't be afraid to add some chia seeds or a handful of nuts to your salad.

But there's still more! Minerals and vitamins are essential for sustaining the valiant work of your liver. Specifically, B vitamins are the hidden gems your liver requires. They support the metabolism of proteins and lipids, aid in the process of detoxification, and help turn food into energy. These vitamins are present in meat, fish, eggs, whole grains, and legumes. What a formidable group of fighters!

Magnesium and zinc are two other minerals that merit attention. With its involvement in more than 300 enzyme interactions within your body, zinc is like your reliable buddy. It shields your liver from damage and aids in the production of enzymes needed for detoxification. For that unrivalled zinc power, add some oysters, meat, pumpkin seeds, or chickpeas to the mixture.

And last, magnesium—the unsung hero of liver health—is mentioned. Like nothing else, it controls liver enzymes, facilitates detoxification, and combats inflammation. Bananas, avocados, almonds, and spinach are great sources of this wonderful mineral, so include them in your diet and give your liver a pat on the back.

Let's now discuss superfoods. Like the Avengers, these superheroes are prepared to save the day and promote the health of your liver. Let's start with beetroot. In addition to being rich in antioxidants, this tiny gem promotes the formation of bile, which helps with digestion and removes toxins. It may be roasted to make a delicious side dish, juiced, or added to salads. It's like an injection of energy for your liver.

Turmeric is the next superhero on our list. Curcumin, an anti-inflammatory and antioxidant molecule, is present in this spice.

It helps the liver become more detoxified and combats inflammation in the liver. Pour some turmeric into your smoothies, soups, and curries, and watch the wonders happen.

Finally, but most definitely not least, there is garlic, the unsung hero of all recipes. Garlic lowers inflammation, promotes detoxification, and activates liver enzymes. It also gives any food a taste boost. Speak about a win-win circumstance.

Yet we must not undervalue the significance of a well-balanced diet. Like the foundation of your liver's army, whole foods are. They offer a variety of nutrients that are beneficial to your general health. You should eat a diet rich in fruits, vegetables, whole grains, lean meats, and healthy fats. Your liver will appreciate the harmonic symphony of flavours and nutrients that they produce together.

That's all there is to it, friend. The best way to combat hepatitis E is to fuel your body with nourishment. You can take charge of your health, strengthen your immune system, and provide your liver with the support it needs by exploring the world of nutrients that are good for your liver. Never forget to raise your antioxidant intake, utilise the power of superfoods, and serve a cuisine that is well-balanced and composed of whole foods. By working together, we can defeat Hepatitis E and take it to task.

Unmasking the Impact of Stress

My friend, let me tell you something. I've felt it in my bones and seen it with my own eyes. Your liver can be severely damaged by stress, and I mean severely. You see, your body releases stress chemicals like cortisol when you're under stress, and chronic stress is like a tornado tearing through your liver. The liver is responsible for several vital functions, including metabolism, detoxification, and hormone regulation. However, when it is constantly exposed to high cortisol levels, it begins to swell and become inflamed, much like a balloon that is about to burst.

A study that was published in Psychoneuroendocrinology provided some insight into the extent to which long-term stress can damage the liver. Researchers discovered that all of these indicators of inflammation and liver damage were present in those who experienced ongoing stress. Even worse, they discovered that stress may exacerbate pre-existing liver diseases like hepatitis E. My friend, stress seems to throw a monkey wrench into the workings of your liver.

But there is hope, I assure you. I have personal experience as a health and wellness coach with the benefits of stress management for the liver. It all comes down to self-care, awareness, and meditation. You know, the small things that bring you inner peace. Being aware is living in the present moment without worry or judgement. It's as like you know what's making you anxious and know how to handle it without losing your composure. A study published in Liver International demonstrated the real impact that mindfulness training can have on liver function. Researchers found that those who engaged in mindfulness practises had reduced liver enzyme levels and experienced reduced levels of anxiety and depression. Thus, my friend, it's a win-win situation.

An additional method for reducing stress is meditation. It's similar like releasing all of your tension and anxiety and plunging into a tranquil pool. It's as though you discover a secret haven of calm in your mind when you concentrate on your breathing or a mantra. And you know what? According to studies, meditation is beneficial for your liver as well. Regular meditation has been shown in gastroenterology to reduce stiffness associated with liver fibrosis. It has also been observed in Psychosomatic Medicine that meditation can even lower those undesirable inflammatory markers in the liver. Thus, my friend, meditation is like armour for your liver.

However, you know what's actually crucial? looking after oneself. I'm talking healthy nutrition, exercise, and sleep. They resemble the fundamentals of self-care. However, it goes beyond the tangibles. It is all about doing what brings you joy and a sense of aliveness. pastimes, the outdoors, and quality family time. They resemble tiny oasis in the middle of tension. I regularly assist individuals in creating self-care regimens that are tailored to their need and stress levels. We identify their motivators and assist them in making it a top priority, particularly when they are coping with an illness like hepatitis E. Like a road plan to a healthier liver and a more contented life.

Stress is serious business, my buddy, especially when it affects your liver. But there's always a path forward, so don't worry. You can use self-care, mindfulness, and meditation as your secret weapons in this conflict. They can improve your life, help you control your stress, and take care of your liver. It's similar to taking charge of your wellbeing and transforming stress into strength. So, my friend, let's get this Hepatitis E problem under control. With the right tools, we can kick stress in the ass.

Exercise: Your Liver's Best Friend

Chapter 6: Exercise: Your Liver's Best Friend

Hi everyone! I practise medicine and coach health and wellness, and I'll tell you that I'm a huge proponent of holistic wellness and healthcare. I work in a field where I have personally witnessed the amazing benefits of exercise in the management of Hepatitis E. I want to reveal to you today the unrealized potential that exists inside the transformational force of exercise.

Now, it's no secret that exercise is the key to excellent health. It's been shown to elevate your mood, strengthen your heart, and generally make you feel amazing. However, most individuals are unaware of the fact that exercise can also significantly improve liver health and help manage Hepatitis E.

You must comprehend how Hepatitis E affects the liver in order to fully appreciate the benefits of exercise for those who have the illness. The insidious virus known as hepatitis E mostly affects the liver, resulting in various forms of inflammation and harm to this priceless organ. Serious illnesses such liver fibrosis, cirrhosis, and even liver cancer may develop as a result of this damage over time.

Hold on, don't get into a panic just yet. My friend, hope remains. Numerous scientific research have demonstrated the beneficial effects of regular physical exercise on the liver and the significant reduction of disease progression risk in individuals with Hepatitis E. Exercise has the incredible power to increase the synthesis of detoxifying enzymes, promote liver regeneration, and enhance liver blood flow.

Allow me to brief you on a fascinating study that was carried out at the University of California, San Francisco. In this study, participants with Hepatitis E were given a regimented exercise programme to follow. The outcomes were astounding. Not only did their liver fibrosis ratings improve, but their liver enzyme levels also decreased, suggesting a reduction in liver inflammation. How about hitting the ball out of the park!

Now, why does physical activity benefit your liver so much? It all comes down to boosting your immune system and generally improving your health. Your body produces more natural killer cells and T-cells, which are incredibly effective at fending off viral infections, when you exercise vigorously.

It gets better, so cling on tightly. An further benefit of regular exercise is a reduction in chronic inflammation, that cunning little devil who loves to wreck havoc on your liver. Not only will you be doing your liver a favour by controlling this inflammation, but you will also be laying the groundwork for a body that is generally healthier. Win-win!

After discussing the scientific aspect, let's move on to the practical side of things. How can you truly include exercise in your life to take care of your liver, which needs it badly? Remember that your workout regimen should be customised for you based on your unique requirements and physical capabilities. Since each person's road to optimal liver health is different, there is no one-size-fits-all method to follow here.

Don't worry if you're just getting started or if your movement is restricted! Exercises with little impact, like tai chi or yoga, may be ideal. These easy workouts improve your general well-being, increase your flexibility, and promote relaxation. They are also adaptable to your specific demands, so people of all fitness levels can use them.

But hold on, I have something special in store for those of you seeking a challenge and a significant improvement in liver health. We refer to it as high-intensity interval training, or HIIT. Here's how it works: you exert yourself for brief intervals of time with high intensity exercise, and then you take rest or lower intensity intervals to catch your breath. This intense exercise programme has been shown to increase insulin resistance, decrease stubborn liver fat, and support your liver.

Finding a fitness regimen that you can stick to and enjoy is crucial in this situation. It's about using movement to unlock your body's incredible healing potential rather than making yourself do something you detest. So, select something that excites you and dedicate yourself to it on a daily basis, regardless of whether you're a sports enthusiast, a dance queen, a water baby, or a hiking enthusiast. Exercise is not a chore, I assure you. It's your go-to tool for transforming your liver health to its best possible state. Your liver is going to be praising you.

That's it for now! The finest thing you can do for your liver is exercise. It has the ability to activate your liver, boost your immune system, and reduce the chance that your Hepatitis E may worsen. There is an exercise programme out there that's ideal for you, ranging from easy yoga stretches to intense high-intensity interval training sessions. Put on your sneakers, turn on your go-to workout music, and let's start this incredible trip together. Your liver will be very appreciative to you.

Nutrition: Fueling Your Liver for Success

Our liver is really something else, you know. It resembles this incredibly strong organ that is capable of self-repair and regeneration. However, it seems that the Hepatitis E virus needs all the assistance it can get. Fortunately for us, there are several nutrients that can help our liver work at its peak and accelerate the healing process. Now let's examine a few of these foods that are good for the liver and learn more about how they function.

Let's start with these fruits that are high in antioxidants. Berries, citrus fruits, and juicy grapes come to mind. These tiny creatures are incredibly rich in substances known as antioxidants, which work to counteract all of the damaging free radicals that are present in our bodies. And antioxidants are crucial when it comes to Hepatitis E! In fact, they can offset all of the oxidative stress brought on by the virus. Thus, by include these fruits in your diet, you're essentially giving your liver the tools it needs to combat the infection and reduce bothersome inflammation.

And these vegetables that help with detoxification. We're talking about cruciferous vegetables, leafy greens, and reliable garlic. These terrible fellas are the closest companions to your liver. They aid in your body's natural detoxification processes and aid in the removal of all pollutants. You should also definitely be careful with your liver when it comes to Hepatitis E. Avoid overdosing it with substances that can exacerbate the situation. Put some vegetables on your plate and allow them to aid in the detoxification process, improving the general health of your liver.

Let's not overlook the fatty fish at this point. Your liver adores the abundance of omega-3 fatty acids found in fish like salmon, mackerel, and sardines. These good fats not only help your liver grow and repair its cells, but they also have wonderful anti-inflammatory qualities that can dramatically reduce liver inflammation. Therefore, by include these fatty fish in your diet, you're essentially providing your liver with everything it needs to repair and regenerate itself. Wow, what a win-win scenario!

Finally, there are these whole grains. Brown rice, quinoa, and oats are like the unsung heroes of liver health. They are a great source of complex carbs and fibre, which assist to balance blood sugar and prevent insulin spikes. That's equivalent to a major liver problem. Furthermore, the presence of these whole grains provides your liver with vital nutrients including magnesium and B vitamins. Therefore, the next time you grab for some grains, give up on the refined varieties and go for the full thing. Your liver will be appreciative!

Naturally, proteins are an important consideration. The components of lean meats, poultry, tofu, and legumes are what your liver needs to heal and regenerate. However, and this is a very important but, choose lean protein sources to spare your liver. As an added bonus, legumes like chickpeas and lentils are a great source of fibre. You you aware of the effects of fibre? It promotes the general health of your liver and helps with digestion. Thus, add these proteins to your diet that are good for your liver and watch it dance.

This brings us to the harsh reality. If you wish to give your liver the upper hand, there are several meals you must limit or completely avoid. The bad guys of the liver world are processed foods, sugary snacks, alcohol, and fried foods. Particularly alcohol may seriously harm your liver, and believe me when I say that the last thing you want when you have Hepatitis E is that. So, reduce your intake of these unhealthy meals as a favour to yourself. Make your liver feel loved so that it can mend.

Okay, so we've covered a lot of territory, but it's time to actually apply what we've learned. I'll be sharing some helpful hints and delicious recipes in the next section to encourage you to make those healthy dietary adjustments. These recipes, which range from tasty stir-fries to smoothies full of nutrients, are not only delicious but also specifically designed to meet the dietary requirements of those living with Hepatitis E. Each one has been thoughtfully designed to maximise the benefits of those components that support the liver. Prepare to fuel your body and adopt a wholistic approach to your recuperation process.

Ultimately, we must not undervalue the significance of nutrition in supporting our recuperation from Hepatitis E. We can help our liver repair and perform at its peak by include items that are good for it in our diet. We can truly take charge of our liver health now that we are well-informed on the advantages of foods that are good for our livers and how to choose them. So let's get started on this healing journey together by devouring those delectable foods and diving into those helpful tips. We can do this!

Stress Less, Live More

Allow me to share a tale with you about Sarah, one of my patients. She was a thirty-something lady leading a busy life with a demanding career, a family to support, and the additional burden of managing her Hepatitis E diagnosis. Sarah sought my advice on how to better take care of her liver and effectively manage her symptoms.

It was evident from our talk that Sarah's health was suffering from stress. She was inundated with worries about her family, career, and health all the time. She didn't seem to ever give herself permission to unwind and look after herself.

I gave Sarah an explanation of how long-term stress affects the liver. Our bodies release cortisol and other stress-related hormones, which might weaken our immune systems. As a result, the liver has a tougher time fending off viruses and illnesses like hepatitis E. Inflammation brought on by stress can also impair the liver's ability to operate. Finally, stress exacerbates the Hepatitis E symptoms.

Sarah's narrative is not unique. Similar difficulties are faced by many patients with chronic disorders such as hepatitis E. Therefore, reducing stress is an essential component of managing hepatitis E.

I offer readers in my book useful techniques for recognising and controlling stressors. Self-awareness is essential because it allows us to lessen the effects of stress by identifying what causes it. Journaling, therapy, and self-reflection activities can all assist us in understanding our emotional triggers.

Building resilience is the next step after identifying our stressors. Being resilient means having the capacity to recover from stress and misfortune. It calls for preserving our good relationships and tending to our emotional wellbeing. I provide a thorough manual on building coping strategies and resilience to effectively manage the difficulties associated with Hepatitis E in my book.

I also go into methods for lowering stress that have been shown to help people relax and de-stress. Yoga, mindfulness meditation, deep breathing techniques, and mild physical activities like tai chi or qigong can all help lower stress levels, strengthen the liver, and promote general wellbeing.

However, I am aware that there is no one-size-fits-all strategy for stress reduction. For this reason, I research complementary and alternative forms of self-care such as massage therapy, acupuncture, herbal supplements, and aromatherapy. Finding comprehensive and successful strategies to reduce stress and enhance liver health while taking culture and personal preferences into account is the aim.

I provide relatable experiences from patients I've treated throughout my book. These inspiring tales demonstrate the beneficial effects of stress reduction on liver health and general well-being. Readers will be encouraged and inspired to apply these tactics in their own lives by showcasing these success stories.

Readers will witness a major shift in their general well-being as well as improvements in their liver health as they learn the art of stress management. They will grow more in sync with their body and emotions, which will enable them to react resiliently and nimbly to stressful situations. Even with Hepatitis E, they will be able to have more balanced and satisfying lives thanks to their enhanced ability to manage stress.

In summary, long-term stress negatively affects liver function and can make it more difficult to treat Hepatitis E. But people can enhance their general well-being and liver health by recognising and controlling their stress triggers, building resilience, and implementing stress-reduction strategies. Readers will set out on a transformative journey towards stress reduction with the tools and tactics I teach in this book, allowing them to enjoy life to the fullest, even in the face of Hepatitis E.

Exercise: Moving Towards Healing

Folks, let me tell you something. Working out is like having a secret weapon against hepatitis E. It's important to give your liver the love it needs to kick some major virus ass, not simply to stretch those muscles and get in shape. I'm talking about cleansing that liver like it's no big deal, lowering inflammation, and enhancing blood flow. Believe me when I say that exercise is key to managing Hepatitis E.

Exercise is one of the most remarkable things because it directly addresses liver inflammation. You know, inflammation is the main symptom of hepatitis E, and it can be very harmful. Now, though, what? In fact, regular exercise can reduce the inflammatory-promoting chemicals' production. It's similar to donning a superhero cape made of natural anti-inflammatory liver tissue. Bid adieu to inflammation in your liver and welcome to a happy, healthier liver.

But friends, that's not all. Exercise is really beneficial for liver fibrosis as well. Now, I realise that the term "fibrosis" seems like science fiction, but in essence, it refers to an accumulation of scar tissue in the liver. Furthermore, if that scar tissue continues to grow, it may result in cirrhosis, a terrible disease that impairs the function of your liver. But worry not—exercise is here to turn things around. Exercise can actually stop the progression of liver fibrosis or even reverse it, according to studies. It resembles going back in time with liver damage. That, in my opinion, is a winning tactic.

This is where the true magic happens, people: in cardio. I mean physical activities that get your heart rate up and your lungs firing, like swimming, cycling, or jogging. Know what that implies, please? It translates to your body receiving nutrients and oxygen like a Ferrari on the Autobahn. What direction do you believe they're going? Yes, directly into your liver. Your liver is receiving all the nourishment it needs to function properly and heal all those injured cells. Cardio also functions as a whole body tune-up. Your cardiovascular system as a whole receives a significant boost, your heart becomes stronger, and your cholesterol levels decrease. And believe me, people, everyone who has Hepatitis E needs it.

Hey, people, let's not overlook strength training. You know, working those muscles hard by lifting those weights or utilising resistance bands. It's not just about wanting to look like a Greek god or goddess—though, let's face it, who wouldn't want that?); it's also about strengthening your body and putting it in peak condition. The best thing is that as you gain muscle mass, your body becomes more insulin-sensitive and your metabolism increases dramatically. And for anyone suffering from liver illness, that, my friends, is music to their ears. In addition, you'll be less likely to fall and stronger and more nimble. Folks, it's win-win.

You must now take it nice and steady when it comes to going back into the fitness routine when you have Hepatitis E. Don't get crazy and begin running full marathons at once. Begin with low-impact exercises like mild yoga or a leisurely stroll. In this manner, you can gradually increase your stamina and ease into the workout regimen. The secret is to follow the American Heart Association's recommendation and aim for at least 150 minutes of moderate-intensity exercise per week. Hey, people, pay attention to your bodies. It's quite acceptable if you need to take it easy one day. Just make sure you quickly get back on course.

People, I have to tell you that in all the years that I have been serving people with Hepatitis E, I have witnessed some amazing changes brought about by exercise. Consider my friend John as an example. He felt disappointed and worn out when he initially learned that he had Hepatitis E. However, after I put him on a customised workout regimen that included cardio, strength training, and stretching, his energy level skyrocketed. All of a sudden, he felt in charge of his health and prepared to face the world.

And there's my friend Sarah. She had been fighting chronic E. coli for what seemed like an eternity. Her medications weren't working very well, and she was depressed. But something amazing happened when she began to incorporate regular exercise into her daily regimen. She felt like a completely different person, her liver inflammation decreased, and her general health improved. She possessed greater cerebral, emotional, and physical strength. People, talk about a whole makeover.

Let's not forget, though, that exercising should always be done under a doctor's supervision and carefully. You must ensure that your fitness regimen is customised to your requirements and physical constraints. Talk to your physician or a certified fitness instructor to make sure you're headed in the right direction. Naturally, it's much more crucial to seek the all-clear from your doctor before beginning an intense exercise regimen if you have a major liver condition or other health problems.

Exercise is ultimately the key to controlling Hepatitis E and maintaining a healthy liver, people. It effectively detoxifies, decreases inflammation, and enhances blood flow. Thus, ensure that you include regular physical exercise in your daily regimen, regardless of whether you like strength training, cardio, or a combination of the two. Believe me, each step you take toward physical activity is a step toward recovery and regaining control over your Hepatitis E experience. Now go forth and take the infection to task!

The Power of Exercise

Unleashing the Healing Power Within

It's funny how, when it comes to healing, we always search outside for answers and remedies. We go through medical procedures, take medication, and have faith that something will heal us. However, what if I told you that we all possess the ability to heal? In my profession, I have personally witnessed it, and let me tell you, it is astounding.

Let's now discuss workout. I'm not only referring to working up a sweat and controlling your affections. Working out is similar to having a magic key that lets our bodies mend themselves. It's like a superpower that intervenes to keep our thoughts sharp and our hearts racing while still maintaining control over our weight.

Imagine yourself out there, swimming to your heart's content, pounding the streets, or twisting into a pretzel during a yoga session. Your body begins to release endorphins, which are these incredible hormones. These natural mood enhancers and pain relievers give you an amazing sense of exhilaration that's sometimes referred to as the "runner's high." And believe me when I say that it's revolutionary. These endorphins not only make you feel amazing, but they also aid in stress reduction and pain relief. Exercise has two beneficial effects at once.

But there's still more! Our immune systems are prepared for battle by exercise. Studies reveal that exercise activates natural killer cells and lymphocytes, which are immune cells that are prepared to fight against infections and diseases. It's similar to deploying the armed forces to protect our bodies. And exercise is the reason for all of this.

So how precisely can exercise boost our defences against disease? Well, inflammation and physical exertion have a lovely tango together. Our bodies are under stress when we exercise, which results in microscopic tears to our muscles and tissues. "Out with the old, in with the new" is a saying that is well-known. Therefore, when a crime occurs, our bodies send out signals to attract immune cells to the area. Immune cells arrive as at a party and tidy up the debris. Furthermore, exercise helps our bodies acquire the oxygen and blood they need to function properly, boosting immunity and eliminating waste.

But, I must emphasise that moderation is essential. In fact, overdoing it or pushing ourselves too hard might exacerbate inflammation and impede the healing process. It all comes down to honouring our boundaries and paying attention to what our bodies are telling us. Rest certain, there exists a thin boundary between pushing ourselves to the limit and exceeding it. Discover your sweet spot and let exercise to do its magic.

The best part is that exercise boosts our general health and wellbeing in addition to boosting our immune systems. Better sleep, reduced stress, and sharper minds are the results. It's like accomplishing all those health objectives at once. Hey, let's not overlook our blood pressure and hearts. They stay happy and healthy when they exercise.

What then is the key to releasing this incredible healing force that resides inside each of us? It's a comprehensive strategy. It's important to embrace all facets of our health and take a broad view. This entails monitoring our diets, controlling our stress levels, and engaging in some good ol' self-care. When you combine these lifestyle modifications with exercise, you have a surefire prescription for overall recovery and wellbeing.

It's nothing short of astounding to witness the amazing transformations that exercise brings about in the lives of my patients. Every one of us possesses a hidden power that is just waiting to be released. So, why do you hesitate? Set modest but attainable goals at first, then push yourself bit by bit. Enjoy the process and pay attention to what your body is trying to tell you. Allow exercise to become a source of happiness, strength, and healing for you.

Finally, let me say that we all possess the amazing ability to heal ourselves. And you know what? The trick is to exercise. It boosts our general wellbeing, releases those endorphins, and prepares our immune system for combat. It's a comprehensive strategy that addresses more than simply physical wellness. So trust in the transformational potential of physical activity. You are more capable than you may realise. Now is the time to realise your capacity for healing.

A Dance With Endorphins

Do you know those tiny compounds in your body that give you a cosy, fuzzy feeling inside? Yes, the chemicals known as endorphins. It appears that they are the key to both feeling well and avoiding suffering. It seems as though our bodies are equipped with innate superheroes who come to our aid when we are in pain or experiencing despair.

It has always been obvious that exercise is good for you, but what's even more amazing is that it raises endorphin levels. Whether it's a brisk walk or an insanely strenuous workout, getting our bodies moving triggers a series of events inside of us that would make even the most scien-fi nerd proud.

Imagine yourself pushing yourself to the limit and feeling the burn when all of a sudden, a tidal wave of positive feelings and endorphins overwhelm your brain. Your body seems to be saying, "Hey, good work! I'll continue to send positive energy your way if you continue." And wow, those vibes really help to push worry and tension behind.

As you can see, stress causes our bodies to release the hormone cortisol, which can have negative effects on both our mental and physical health. However, when we exercise and produce those endorphins, it feels as though we're taking a relaxing drug straight out of nature's pharmacy. All of a sudden, the world becomes much lighter, and a feeling of calm descends upon us like a warm blanket.

But things get very fantastic from here on out. Not only do endorphins improve our mental health, but they are also highly effective pain relievers. They essentially turn off the pain signals that are begging for attention when they attach themselves to receptors in our brains. It functions as a natural, non-addictive switch to turn off pain.

It makes sense why exercise is regarded as the best way to improve mood and reduce stress. It feels like we've reached a completely new level of joy and that everything around us is now brimming with vibrancy and colour. Furthermore, it extends far beyond mental health. Frequent exercise can increase our self-esteem and shield us from the worst effects of anxiety and melancholy.

Imagine yourself feeling like you're on top of the world as you perform your joyful dance and feel the music coursing through your veins. The energy spike and perspiration on your forehead are indicators that endorphins are working hard to give you a sense of invincibility.

So how can one get this power? Discover a passion or hobby that you can persist with. It may be doing yoga in your living room, hitting the pavement, or swaying back and forth on the dance floor. Simply start moving and allow your heart rate to rise. Observe how your body responds, welcome the rush, and allow the music to lead you to your happy place.

Recall that this is a journey. Begin small, make incremental progress, and observe as you push over your comfort zone and accomplish goals you never would have imagined. Treat yourself with respect, pay attention to your body's demands, and acknowledge each small accomplishment as it comes along.

There are no limitations or walls in the universe of endorphins. The benefits are limitless and the possibilities are unlimited. So grab a pair of dancing shoes, turn up the music, and prepare to have the time of your life as those feel-good hormones take you. Dancing will lead you to a place of happiness, ecstasy, and constant wellbeing.

Reviving the Liver With Movement

The liver is essentially our body's unsung hero. It plays an incredibly significant function in maintaining our health and well-being. It creates lipids and proteins, regulates our metabolism, and detoxifies everything we put into our bodies. However, when things go wrong and the liver becomes damaged, as happens when Hepatitis E strikes, it is no longer able to function as it should. And that's where it comes, my friend, from exercising.

Here's the thing: studies have shown that exercise improves liver health in addition to heart health. Exercise causes our blood vessels to dilate and our heart to beat more quickly, allowing blood to flow freely throughout our bodies, including the liver. Because of this increase in blood flow, the liver is able to detoxify substances more successfully and receives more oxygen and minerals. How about boosting the energy in your liver?

That's not all, though. In fact, studies have shown that exercise can help lessen inflammation and the undesirable accumulation of liver fat. As you can see, these are major causes of liver disorders, such as non-alcoholic fatty liver disease. You can therefore bid farewell to extra liver fat and hello to a healthier liver by getting off the couch and taking action. How fantastic is that?

What form of physical activity is best for your liver right now? It all comes down to striking a balance between strengthening your muscles and raising your heart rate. To raise your heart rate, consider engaging in physical activities like cycling, swimming, jogging, or brisk walking. Remember to practise resistance training as well! That's the thing that keeps your body functioning normally and aids in muscular growth. It functions for your liver health as a tag team pair.

Experts advise aiming for two or more strength training sessions and at least 150 minutes of moderate-intensity aerobic activity per week. I assure you that this combination will not only revitalise your liver but also improve your overall well-being.

But hold on, it's a good idea to see your doctor or a fitness expert before diving headfirst into a new exercise regimen. You don't want to screw things up, especially if you have Hepatitis E or any other health problems. They will assist you in determining the ideal fitness regimen for you and ensure your safety.

Now pay attention! It is necessary to exercise with a little more caution if you have Hepatitis E. Go cautiously and slowly, my friend. You don't want to put yourself through unnecessary stress or discomfort. Rather than taxing the liver, we wish to aid in its repair. Hence, begin slowly and increase your speed. And be careful to reduce dosage a little if you experience any pain. No worries, we've got this!

Hey, it's not all about those intense workouts that make you sweat. Other exercises and routines can help show your liver some additional care. Consider doing qigong, yoga, or tai chi. These are all about those soft, flowing motions that can help you discover your zen, lower stress levels, and increase blood flow. My friend, that's not all. Exercises for flexibility and stretching can also be quite beneficial. Thus, roll out those shoulders, perform some side bends, and extend your calves. The newly drawn blood that is oxygenated will be much appreciated by your liver.

But remember, physical activity is only one piece of the jigsaw when it comes to eradicating Hepatitis E. You need to control your stress levels, watch what you eat, and get enough beauty sleep. You know, it's all about that all-encompassing attitude. Your liver will have the best chance of healing and recovering if you take care of everything.

In summary, exercise is the key to rejuvenating your liver and restoring its optimal function. It increases blood flow, facilitates detoxifying, and eliminates liver fat. Strike a balance between strength and aerobic training, add some easy motions and stretches, and don't forget to look after your general health. You'll be showing Hepatitis E who's boss in no time with the correct actions and lifestyle adjustments, I promise.

The Immune Booster Workout

Now that we've covered it, let's speak about how exercise can significantly strengthen your immune system. Yes, you did hear correctly. When it comes to warding off infections, working out and sweating it out are revolutionary. Who would have guessed that a great workout could help you fortify yourself against a virus like hepatitis E?

However, we must warm up before getting into the specifics of this immune-boosting exercise. Imagine it as a gentle transition into a steaming bath or as a morning stretch for those sore joints. Your body needs to be prepared for action. I mean a good five to ten minutes of light aerobic exercise, such as brisk walking or vigorous cycling. Your core temperature rises as a result, warming up your muscles and preparing them for action.

Let's now move on to the enjoyable part: strength training. This is an essential component of the immune-boosting regimen. You'll be strengthening your entire strength, gaining muscle, and enhancing your balance. And you know what? Your immune cells get activated and prepared for action. We're talking about planks, push-ups, lunges, and squats. If you've never lifted weights before, start off small and work your way up. Hey, don't forget about proper form. We wish to train our immune army without any injuries interfering.

But hold on, we're not quite done. Exercise for the heart. This is your pass to better lung function and a more robust cardiovascular system. It's similar to sending your immune cells on a fast express train to their destination. There are several options available here. Go crazy and run, swim, dance, cycle, and jump rope. Simply try to get in at least 30 minutes most days of the week, and you'll see your immune system transform into a superhero.

Let's switch it up now and incorporate some zen into this exercise. Flexibility and serenity are not the only benefits of yoga and mind-body exercises. In fact, they also strengthen your immune system. Crazy, you say? So why not give some Pilates, Tai Chi, or yoga poses a try? With increased balance, flexibility, and decreased stress, you're essentially building an immune-blasting machine.

It's time to stretch and cool down after your incredible workout while you're all fired up. Friends, don't skip this section. Restoring your heart rate to normal and eliminating any impurities in your system can be achieved with a 5- to 10-minute mild cycling or jogging session. Oh, and don't overlook the stretching exercises. Aim for 15 to 30 seconds of holding each stretch, concentrating on the main muscle groups. I promise it will increase your range of motion, release stress, and prepare you for your next immune-boosting adventure.

That concludes the greatest immune-boosting exercise. Your immune system is receiving the care it needs when you include strength training, cardio, yoga, and a thorough cool-down. Remain steady, increase the intensity little by little, and pay attention to your body at all times. And don't be afraid to ask a fitness expert for advice if you need it.

Now, fellow fighters, let's take on Hepatitis E with an immune-boosting workout! Let's maximise movement, sweat, and empowerment. Prepare to kick some assholes!

Finding Joy in Movement

I have always found the profound relationship between our bodies and minds to be absolutely fascinating. Our ideas, feelings, and experiences seem to be entwined with every strand of our bodily being. However, that relationship becomes even more astounding when it comes to mobility.

I will always remember this particular patient, Jessica. She sought my assistance because she was experiencing ongoing weariness and emotional exhaustion. She was psychologically exhausted from the long hours she had to spend at her desk in the corporate world. Imagine being caught in a repetitive cycle of work, sleep, and so on. She yearned for some passion, spontaneity, and happiness in her life.

It hit me like a tonne of bricks as we looked into Jessica's predicament in more detail. Her emotional discomfort was essentially being fueled by her inactive lifestyle. She didn't have any movement whatsoever throughout her life. She was hooked to her chair for the majority of her waking hours and had denied herself the simple joy of doing physical things that ignited her soul.

The issue is, though, Jessica genuinely wanted things to be different. She simply lacked the drive to make exercise a part of her everyday schedule. Instead of seeing exercise as an opportunity for self-expression and self-discovery, she saw it as a terrible burden and obligation. That insight got me to thinking: perhaps I ought to tell her stories that could inspire her in the same way.

I began by telling her about John, a middle-aged man who used movement to dramatically change his life. He felt lost and cut off from everything and everyone around him due to depression and addiction. But what did he do, you know? He made the decision to just go for daily walks.

Now, John had difficulty at first. He took brief hikes that had no real significance or goal. But as he continued to walk, something amazing occurred: he rediscovering a sense of exhilaration and freedom he had long since lost. He started using walking as a kind of meditation and self-connection with the natural world. He immediately began experimenting with different types of movement, such as yoga and dancing. His lifeline was movement, which helped him emerge from the shadowy abyss and into a vibrant, purpose-filled life.

Motivated and inspired by John's narrative, Jessica set out to investigate various types of movement on her own. She tried dancing, Pilates, and yoga, appreciating the mental and physical health benefits of each discipline. And believe me when I say that she revealed layers of happiness that had been hidden inside of her with each stride she made. She began to use movement as a tool of self-discovery and reestablishing her connection to her body, mind, and soul.

I encounter a great deal of folks in my line of work who have just lost their appreciation for movement. They've given up on playfulness and neglected their bodies due to the stresses of adult duties, work-related stress, and daily life constraints. But believe me, no matter your age or level of fitness, you can all rediscover that joy. It all begins with a mental shift, viewing exercise as an exciting chance to express ourselves, develop, and connect rather than as a burden.

You need to identify activities that truly speak to your interests and personality if you want to infuse your workout regimen with passion, purpose, and a little playfulness. What gives you life, you might ask? What makes you happy pure and simple? After that, venture outside and experiment with various movement styles that suit your tastes. The options are unlimited, my buddy, whether you want to swim, go into the bush, dance nonstop, or ride a bike.

The trouble is, though, that identifying the things that light your fire is not the only thing to do. You must approach movement with an open mind and a curious attitude. Give yourself permission to try out various methods and approaches. Accept that you are a beginning with no unrealistic expectations and no self-judgment. Every step you take on the journey of movement is a wonderful opportunity for personal development and self-discovery, my buddy.

You also need to keep in mind that there is more to finding delight in moving than just the actual physical exercise. It also depends on how you go about doing it. You have to embrace your playful side, where you may be fully present and let go of any inhibitions. Run like the wind is blowing you away, dance like no one is watching, and cycle with an exuberant sense of innocent joy. Allow movement to become a natural extension of who you are and a means of revealing your inner happiness.

And you know what? As we go deeper into the upcoming chapters, we'll examine particular methods and approaches that can help you bring a tonne of joy and purpose to your workout regimen. In order to make you fall madly in love with movement and discover your inner joy, we're covering everything from finding a supportive community to incorporating mindfulness into your exercises.

The most crucial thing to remember is that movement is more than just a means to an end. It's a deep, life-changing experience that can improve every area of your existence. So let's embark on this amazing journey together, my friend. Together, let's walk the route that brings more happiness, contentment, and self-awareness. I can assure you that it will be truly spectacular.

The Journey of a Thousand Steps

Hi everyone! I am aware that living with hepatitis E can be difficult, but believe me when I say that making exercise a daily part of your routine will alter your life. It improves your immune system, helps you maintain a healthy weight, and works wonders for your mental health. I understand that beginning an exercise regimen might be scary, particularly if you haven't been active in a long time. But don't worry, dear friend—I'll be by your side every step of the way. We'll work together to make sure your journey to a healthier and fitter lifestyle is an incredible success.

Now, let's get to the point. First and foremost, you must establish reasonable objectives. You need to be honest with yourself about your current situation and your capacity for handling things. Spending time putting yourself in other people's shoes or having irrational expectations will only make you feel dissatisfied and unmotivated. Rather, concentrate on your own development and acknowledge each small victory you encounter along the road.

Finding things that you truly enjoy to do is the enjoyable part now. Whether it's stomping on the dance floor, jumping on a bike, diving into a cool pool, or just enjoying a leisurely stroll in the outdoors, consider what it is that gets you moving. Experiment until you discover the activities that truly resonate with you. Recall that working out ought to be something you actually look forward to and enjoy rather than a duty.

It's time to incorporate fitness into your daily routine when you've found your passions. Schedule those workouts on your calendar in the same way that you would any other significant event. This will assist you in making exercise a priority and guarantee that it becomes an essential component of your daily schedule. Find a routine that works for you, whether that means getting up a bit earlier to go for a morning jog or fitting in a yoga session during your lunch break.

But let's face it, there will be days when you simply don't feel like working out; these are the moments when fatigue and a lack of desire could easily derail you. That's when you need to use your mindset's power. Remind yourself of the benefits of exercise for your health and why it is important to you. Imagine yourself finishing that difficult workout or reaching the finish line. When your motivation wanes, surround yourself with inspiring sayings, positive affirmations, or pictures of your heroes.

Monitoring your advancement is another clever way to maintain motivation. Keep a journal of your workouts, logging the length, intensity, and any personal bests. Not only does it allow you to gauge your progress, but it also serves as a constant reminder of your hard work and devotion. Seeing your progress recorded on paper will keep you motivated and ready to keep going even when things get difficult. It's like getting a boost of adrenaline directly into your veins.

Naturally, there will be challenges in the path. But do not worry, my friend; we have plans to get past those obstacles. Time constraints are a typical barrier, yet even ten minutes of exercise can have an impact. Never undervalue those little spurts of action. If you are unable to set up a long period of time for your workout, divide it up into shorter bursts during the day. Go for a walk during your lunch break, include some squats into your Netflix binge, or use the stairs rather than the elevator. Believe me, every little bit matters.

Another ninja barrier that can threaten to impede your progress is boredom. Regularly following the same workout regimen can turn into a snooze fest. For this reason, you must mix things up to keep things interesting. To add a bit more social connection, try new things, change up the intensity of your workouts, or enrol in a group class. You can even push yourself by setting new objectives and trying out different tools or training methods. My friend, stir things up and don't let up on the enthusiasm.

Physical restrictions and injuries may occasionally also show their ugly heads. Before beginning an exercise regimen, be careful to speak with your healthcare practitioner if you have a medical condition or injury. They will instruct you on safe and appropriate exercises for your particular situation. Keep in mind that every person has a different journey, so pay attention to your body and adjust your workouts as necessary.

My friend, consistency is the key component. It's what turns a productive routine into a reflexive behaviour that eventually results in long-term success. Failures or brief plateaus shouldn't demotivate you. There will always be ups and downs in progress. It's not always a straight line. However, remain dedicated to your objectives, exercise consistently, and have faith in the process. You can do this!

Remember that this amazing journey offers you the chance to grow personally and know more about yourself in addition to experiencing physical transformation. Accept the difficulties and acknowledge each accomplishment, no matter how tiny. You're creating the foundation for a healthier and happier future by taking care of your body, mind, and soul with every step you take forward.

Remember that this is your journey, my friend. You are capable of taking charge of your health and changing your life for the better. It is ultimately your responsibility to take the initial move; I am here to help and advise you.

Now put on your shoes, inhale deeply, and embark on a journey of a thousand steps. Accept the boundless opportunities, maintain consistency, and have faith in yourself. We'll work together to realise your full potential and design a life that is as healthy and fulfilling as possible. Let us proceed!

Coping With Challenges

The Rollercoaster of Emotions

I have to be honest with you, listen. Working as a medical doctor and health and wellness coach, I have experienced some odd things. Furthermore, Hepatitis E is not to be taken lightly. The entire experience is one big emotional roller coaster.

Man, I was really hit hard when I realised I had Hepatitis E. It resembled a tidal surge of uncertainty, despair, and terror. It felt like the earth was being torn out from beneath me, and I was unable to comprehend it. I was left feeling helpless and defenceless, unsure of what was ahead.

But the journey was far from over. Oh no, Mr. It had only barely begun. Dealing with a variety of ups and downs was part of managing hepatitis e. On certain days, I felt like a warrior, prepared to kick this illness in the ass. Optimism and hope were coursing through me. I thought that I could overcome this with the correct care and encouragement. And that optimism served as my rocket fuel, enabling me to move forward, take charge of my health, and fight for what I believed was right.

However, I must admit that there were some very difficult days. Merely the bodily signs were sufficient to bring me to my knees. Abdominal pain, nausea, and fatigue all had an adverse effect on my emotional health. It seemed like I was fighting my body all the time. There were moments when I felt as though despair, rage, and frustration would consume me. You know, all I wanted was a semblance of normalcy.

One thing I had to learn in order to go through this emotional rollercoaster was to take care of yourself, guy. My lifeline became self-care. I needed to unwind, rejuvenate, and discover happiness in the little things. I turned to yoga to reestablish a physical connection with my body and meditation to regain mental calm. Those quiet times felt like little islands in the middle of my journey's tumult.

But I also required assistance. I met a group of folks who understood exactly what I was going through and turned to my loved ones for support. I felt less alone after telling my tale and listening to others' stories. Knowing that I wasn't alone on this crazy journey felt like a weight was lifted off my shoulders.

And you know what gave me a complete makeover? a mental change. I began to view Hepatitis E as a chance for resilience and personal development rather than as this huge obstacle. I came to see how my experience may uplift and improve the lives of others. Man, that gave me a completely new purpose.

I also assist people with Hepatitis E in navigating their own emotional rollercoaster as part of my profession. I provide them with the resources they require to handle the highs and lows. We discuss getting help, managing stress, and practising self-care. In addition to treating the disease's physical symptoms, emotional and psychological issues must also be addressed.

I share all of my personal experiences and knowledge in "The Hepatitis E Mastery Bible: Your Blueprint for Complete Hepatitis E Management." Man, I tell it like it is. I want people to know that they can overcome this emotional rollercoaster and that they're not alone. Together, we can build a life that is thriving, joyful, and full of hope.

Hold on tight. We may be on an uneven journey together, but we're not alone. Let's take on those emotional obstacles head-on and emerge from them stronger. Who's with me now?

Finding Strength in Vulnerability

I'll tell you something: showing vulnerability does not imply being weak. It actually reveals our actual strength, much like a hidden superpower. After treating Hepatitis E patients for years, I can assure you that vulnerability is a game-changer. Those who receive this diagnosis frequently experience feelings of heaviness and isolation. Their emotions are all over the place, and the healthcare system can be a maze. The truth is, though: accepting vulnerability has the power to transform everything.

Let me tell you, I've experienced vulnerability on my own. I used to believe that being a doctor required me to always be strong. I believed that being vulnerable was a sign of weakness and would prevent me from giving my patients the best care possible. However, I was greatly mistaken when I began treating patients who had Hepatitis E. It was important to embrace vulnerability rather than run from it.

Sarah was one of the patients. She was trying to hide her concerns and put on a strong face when I first met her. But the more time we had together, the more I prodded her to be vulnerable. And my, what concerns she had. She was afraid of being looked down upon and of having her loved ones reject her. She experienced an immense burden on her shoulders, pressing her to conceal her illness. But what's the deal? I observed Sarah's power when she opened up. It takes bravery to own up to your anxieties and ask for assistance.

We worked together to help Sarah accept her vulnerability. We introduced her to support groups, which provided her with a platform to interact with like-minded individuals. And believe me when I say that it completely changed her life. She came to the realisation that she wasn't alone and that other people could relate to what she was going through. She created a network of support by accepting her vulnerability, which helped her feel strong and empowered.

My relationship with my patients has evolved as a result of accepting vulnerability. They can open up to me because I've established a safe atmosphere where I share my own weaknesses and challenges. And believe me when I say that: that relationship is crucial. It enables me to offer individualised care that is catered to each person's particular needs.

I have developed a series of reflecting exercises to assist my patients in accepting vulnerability. These activities promote acceptance and self-awareness in oneself. We delve deeply into their feelings, insecurities, and concerns. They also learn about their own perseverance and strength throughout this process.

I really enjoy doing an exercise where people write about their experience living with Hepatitis E. It allows them to take stock of their progress and acknowledge their resilience and improvement. It serves as a reminder that showing vulnerability can lead to personal growth rather than being a sign of weakness.

But what's the deal? It's not only about working out. In addition, I advise my patients to look for further assistance, such as counselling or therapy. They now have the means to deal with the psychological and emotional challenges of having hepatitis E thanks to these resources. They can learn coping skills, explore their feelings, and discover fresh approaches to accepting vulnerability through therapy.

Adopting vulnerability is not a simple task, I promise. It calls on us to get up from our comfort zones and confront our worries. However, I promise it's worthwhile. We can reach our full potential when we choose to be vulnerable. We muster the courage to confront the difficulties posed by hepatitis E with sincerity and resolute determination.

Let's embrace our vulnerability, my friends. Together, we can overcome our insecurities, face our fears, and realise our full potential. Let's apply all of our strength to meet the problems posed by hepatitis E. Because vulnerability ultimately presents a chance for development and resilience rather than being a sign of weakness. And I firmly think that we possess the capabilities to conquer any obstacle that may arise.

Navigating the Dark Days

Let me tell you, having Hepatitis E is not an easy life. It feels as though your body and emotions are being struck twice. I know because I've witnessed so many others go through these difficult times that it negatively impacts mental health. The physical symptoms alone, such as exhaustion, nausea, and muscle aches, can knock you out cold and make you want to curl up in bed forever. It becomes even more daunting when you factor in the emotional rollercoaster of stress, worry, and despair.

But, my friend, here's the thing. There are strategies to get through these difficult moments. Although it's not simple, you can take back control of your life if you're prepared to work for it. Accepting your reality and acknowledging it is the first step. Yes, that is awful. It is depressing. It irritates me. And feeling all of those emotions is acceptable. Even if your life was only briefly gone, you must give yourself permission to mourn for the life you once had. Permit yourself to be sad and to lament the things you can no longer do on bad days. Every step of the healing process involves it.

It's time to prioritise self-care when you've come to terms with your situation. You know, looking after your bodily and mental needs. You have to create a routine around the things that make you happy and comfortable. Perhaps you should take a long, relaxing soak in the tub or do some light stretches to keep your body moving. Alternatively, it could be engaging in a creative pastime as a kind of distraction. Make it a regular part of your life, whatever it may be. And never forget that taking care of yourself is not selfish. It's an essential self-defense mechanism.

Apart from taking care of yourself, you also need to learn coping skills. These are the tips you can carry with you to help you deal with the highs and lows of having hepatitis E. Since each of us is unique, your coping mechanism may differ from mine. However, there are certain things that most individuals find effective. Practices for deep breathing can help reduce tension and anxiety. Finding some calm throughout the storm can be facilitated by mindfulness and meditation. Putting your feelings down on paper through journaling is a terrific technique to release those feelings. Additionally, keep in mind the influence of support. Remind yourself that you're not travelling alone by having a conversation with your loved ones or joining a support group.

Let's now discuss your diet. You need to watch what you eat since hepatitis E might cause intestinal problems. To create a diet plan that suits you, it's a good idea to consult a nutritionist or healthcare provider. Overall though, make an effort to prioritise nutrient-dense foods such as whole grains, fruits, vegetables, and lean proteins. Remember to remain hydrated as well. You should drink lots of water and limit your intake of alcohol and caffeine as hepatitis E can cause dehydration.

I understand that you're exhausted, but bear with me. My friend, exercise is essential. Moving around can help your body and mind, even though I know it might be difficult when you're feeling so exhausted. Commence with mild exercises such as strolling, swimming, or doing yoga. Exercise releases endorphins, which are essentially organic mood enhancers. And who knows, they might even assist to reduce tiredness.

We must not overlook your psychological well-being. Feeling melancholy, nervous, or even sad at this time is quite natural. If you need therapy or counselling, don't be scared to get help. You can process those feelings and acquire coping mechanisms for handling stress and uncertainty by speaking with a qualified specialist. And hey, to keep your thoughts focused on the good even in the face of gloomy circumstances, try repeating these positive affirmations and visualisation exercises.

Finally, understand that the process of healing is not linear. It's certain that you will experience both good and bad days. Everything is a part of the process. Thus, remember to treat yourself with kindness when things are difficult. Rely on your network of family, friends, and medical professionals. In the face of Hepatitis E, you can discover resilience and strength in one another.

Now, dear friend, inhale deeply. Although it's challenging, we can succeed. We are capable of navigating through these difficult times, and we will eventually find our way back to the light. There's always someone willing to help, so you're not alone in this.

Adapting to a New Normal

Let me tell you, having Hepatitis E is like entering a completely different planet. It completely upends and changes your daily existence. All of a sudden, the activities you used to perform without giving them any thought turn into a deliberate dance of physical adaptation. I won't deny that it's overwhelming, but I'm here to assist you navigate this wild ride and establish yourself in this new normal.

Your diet is going to be one of the first things you need to consider. Your liver is like your body's own self-cleaning oven when you have hepatitis E. Everything we pour into it is broken down and detoxified by it. It follows that we should provide that poor liver with more care. Believe me when I say that altering my diet significantly helped to manage my symptoms and encourage healing during my personal Hepatitis E battle.

The bottom line is that you need to consume fewer processed and high-fat foods. It's like asking a child not to eat candy, I know, I know. But let me explain. These meals slow down your liver's healing process and increase its stress levels. Rather, concentrate on packing your diet full of complete, high-nutrient foods. Consider lean proteins, whole grains, fruits, and veggies. These nasty boys are loaded with antioxidants, vitamins, and minerals that support the function of your liver and your body as a whole.

And speaking of alcohol, it's time to put it down. My friend, alcohol and livers don't mix. particularly if Hepatitis E is active in your body. Alcohol is harmful to the liver, so adding it to the mix will only make things worse. I understand that giving up alcohol might be difficult. But don't worry, you can get support from a support group or your healthcare professional to help you adjust to your new, alcohol-free lifestyle.

Let's now discuss food planning. It may seem uninteresting, but believe me—it can save your life. Cooking up a storm is the last thing you want to do when you're not feeling your best. Meal planning then becomes important. I'm referring to meal planning so that, regardless of how exhausted or uninspired you are, you always have wholesome options available to you. Hey, enlist the help of a friend or family member instead of doing it alone. It's like a cosy, bonding hobby that fills you with warmth and comfort.

You need to adhere to your medication schedule in addition to all of these dietary adjustments. Depending on how severe your Hepatitis E is, you may be taking immunomodulators or antiviral drugs like crazy. It's critical to follow your doctor's instructions on dosage and scheduling. To help you stay on track, use fancy applications or set reminders on your phone. You should not play around with these material, I assure you.

My friend, let's not overlook the need of self-care. Along this path, self-care is essential. Seek methods for lowering your stress levels, getting some rest, and being active. Physical activity is like having a health superhero. It will support your immune system, lower inflammation, and help you maintain a healthy weight—all of which are critical defences against Hepatitis E. Don't start training for a marathon just yet. Make sure you're selecting the appropriate activity for you by first speaking with your doctor.

The problem is that all of these modifications may give you the impression that you are walking on a thin rope. That's the reason getting counselling and mental support is so crucial. Look for support groups or have a conversation with a therapist who focuses on long-term conditions. It can really transform your life to have a safe place where you can talk about your experiences, pick up new coping mechanisms, and make connections with people who understand you. It's like having a squad that has your back, I promise.

In summary, having hepatitis E shouldn't define or limit who you are. Yes, it will throw you some curveballs, but you underestimate your strength. While adaptation may include altering your routines, it also presents an opportunity for development and fortitude. I can attest to the fact that adopting these lifestyle changes can completely change your life. So go ahead and give self-care first priority, adjust your diet, take your medications as prescribed, get help, and strike that perfect balance. Hepatitis E be damned, you are capable of leading an amazing life that is full of health, happiness, and energy!

My friend, never forget that this is a journey. Be kind with yourself. Every advancement is a success in and of itself. You possess the ability to overcome the obstacles posed by Hepatitis E and lead the greatest possible life. Go forth now and demonstrate your abilities to the world!

The Power of Support

Oh my goodness, it felt like a tonne of bricks when I learned I had Hepatitis E. In an instant, it felt as though my entire universe had been flipped upside down. It's oppressive, you know, the worry and uncertainty that accompany a chronic condition. Fortunately, though, I had a fantastic support network that kind of swooped in and kept me going when I thought I was about to collapse.

Throughout it all, my loved ones, family, and friends have been my superheroes. They surrounded me with their tender love and support, and it really did make a world of difference. They helped me along the entire journey, which gave me the confidence and willpower to face this head-on.

However, you know who truly astounded me? Neha, my younger sister. She has always been my pillar of support. She turned into this incredible encyclopaedia of information about Hepatitis E the instant I received the diagnosis. She most likely knew more about it than my doctor, I promise! She conducted extensive study to learn about the most recent medical procedures and sickness management strategies. She even assisted me with doctor appointments, believe it or not. She was there for me at every turn, asked questions I never would have thought to ask, and took expert notes. Without a doubt, she has been my guardian angel.

It's absurd to imagine that unanticipated sources of support can also provide assistance, you know? I found this Hepatitis E support group by accident, and let me tell you, it changed my life. Going to that first meeting made me scared as hell, but as soon as I walked into the room and saw all these other individuals who understood what I was going through, I felt instantly at ease. We grew close by discussing our dreams, frustrations, and worries. It developed into a secure environment where people could open up and rely on one another. Trust me when I say that having that type of understanding and support is invaluable.

Of course, I also have to consider the medical professionals. I have an obligation to support my fellow medical professionals as a doctor. For me, finding a physician who specialised in Hepatitis E was revolutionary. It was a game-changer to have someone who truly understood what they were talking about, who could break down all the finer points and respond to all of my inquiries. They handled me not just like another patient, but as a person with dreams and worries. Our relationship was founded on trust, and it played a crucial role in my recovery.

Man, creating a support system is not easy. But believe me, it's worthwhile. You need to connect with your loved ones, share your troubles with them, and let them know what's going on. Additionally, don't be hesitant to seek expert assistance; these physicians and specialists are knowledgeable. But you know what, it's powerful to find others who are experiencing similar things. Whether it's in person or online, joining a support group offers you a sense of understanding and community that you just can't get anywhere else.

Hey, remember to look after yourself as well. I started journaling and practising mindfulness, and wow, those two things really helped bring some calm and control to this crazy adventure. Additionally, improving one's diet, increasing physical activity, and lowering stress levels can all have a significant impact on how well this illness is managed. However, it is advisable to seek advice from knowledgeable professionals rather than attempting to handle everything alone.

Living with Hepatitis E is therefore difficult. You don't have to work alone, though. That is essential. Be in the company of kind, understanding, and encouraging individuals. Because, believe me, having their support can make the difference between barely making it through and actually beating this sickness head-on. Thus, cherish that bond, dear friend, cling to it, and face this adventure with poise and fortitude. You can do this.

Embracing Moments of Joy

The significance of savouring those happy moments was particularly brought home to me this one time, as I recall. I was relaxing in my backyard with a cup of tea on a bright morning. There was an explosion of colour in the flowers, and the birds were chirping nonstop. Like, you know, it was like a freaking postcard. I suddenly realised that, despite having to cope with this ridiculous case of Hepatitis E, there were still these small bursts of joy that I could cling to. I was very grateful to have been able to appreciate nature's beauty and find some serenity after coming to that epiphany.

Believe me when I say that one of the best strategies for surviving with hepatitis E is to find happiness in the small successes. It's very simple to become so engrossed in the difficulties and disappointments that you fail to recognise and appreciate your successes, no matter how minor. A good attitude begins to develop when you take the time to genuinely acknowledge and value those small victories, though, as if a switch in your brain flicks. Just following your treatment plan and taking your medications as prescribed could be one of those successes. You win every single day, my buddy, when you obey your doctor's advice. And you get the fortitude and perseverance to take on this Hepatitis E monster head-on because of those tiny successes.

Let's now move on to more realistic topics. I mean, how can one truly wring happiness out of life when confined to a chronic illness? Embracing those times of joy can be greatly enhanced by practising thankfulness, as I have discovered. You may genuinely shift your perspective and concentrate on the positive aspects of life by dedicating a little period of time each day to reflect on your blessings. A nice night's sleep, a supportive word from a loved one, or even just staring at a breathtaking sunset could qualify as simple pleasures.

Happiness can be yours if you can discover those tiny kernels of appreciation in the here and now.

Engaging in joyful and soul-satisfying activities is another beneficial thing. Truly, anything might be the culprit. Something as simple as taking care of yourself, or as complex as devoting yourself to a hobby or interest. Writing brings me a great deal of happiness and calm. It's as like it's my getaway from the actual world. I find this deep sense of contentment because it allows me to express all of my ideas and feelings. You may unleash the power of sickness and embrace your true self, imperfections and all, by discovering and making time for the activities that bring you joy.

It goes beyond pursuing happiness on your own, guy. It is essential that you surround yourself with like-minded people. It makes all the difference in the world to surround yourself with supportive individuals who encourage you and provide a secure environment in which you can share your highs and lows. It seems like an amazing sense of belonging floods over you when you can share those small moments of joy with people who genuinely understand your hardships and triumphs. Your resistance is strengthened, and it provides you with an additional push to press on.

Let us not overlook the affective aspect of the matter, either. Joyfully accepting life does not imply ignoring hardship. It all boils down to striking a balance between seeking out those happy times and facing and tackling the obstacles. For that, seeking professional assistance such as therapy or counselling may be necessary. Alternate therapies may be the solution for helping you better control your stress and improve your mental health. See what works for you, man—everyone is different.

Essentially, my friend, you can encourage yourself and others to discover beauty and happiness even in the midst of Hepatitis E by embracing those times of delight and finding gratitude in the present. There are a lot of things to be grateful for and happy about in life, despite all of its ups and downs, including this silly illness. Life is a priceless gift. Therefore, seize whatever tiny moments of happiness that you may find outside. Your journey to defeating Hepatitis E will be illuminated by them.

Integrative Therapies

The Ancient Art of Acupuncture

Let me tell you, my buddy, acupuncture is very revolutionary. Imagine your body as a complex system of energy channels, akin to an entire highway system, through which the essential energy known as Qi flows. According to traditional Chinese medicine, problems begin to arise and illnesses start to appear one after the other when this Qi becomes completely obstructed or disturbed. But do not worry, acupuncture intervenes to save the day, my friend. By pressing and prodding particular areas along those energy highways, it seeks to restore the Qi balance, which in turn initiates the healing process.

Let's now discuss hepatitis E. According to research, acupuncture can be a very effective treatment for this illness. It is akin to a superpower for your body, enhancing its innate ability to heal, boosting immunity, and boosting your liver. Not convinced by me? A research published in the Journal of Traditional Chinese Medicine revealed that people with chronic hepatitis could legitimately lower their liver enzyme levels using acupuncture. And get this: in patients with chronic hepatitis B, acupuncture plus antiviral therapy boosted the rate of viral clearance, according to a second study published in the World Journal of Gastroenterology. That's what I refer to as a double dose of goodness.

Acupuncture not only supports your liver, but it also alleviates the bothersome symptoms associated with Hepatitis E. You are aware of the weariness, nausea, and pain in the abdomen. It resembles a magic act. Your soreness will disappear once the needles are inserted into your body's hidden pressure points, which produce endorphins, which are natural painkillers. But there's still more. Additionally, acupuncture helps to regulate your digestive system, curb inflammation, and enhance your general health. In essence, it makes you feel amazing, and who wouldn't want that?

But the actual deal is this. Not only does acupuncture treat physical ailments, but it also has a profound effect on mental and emotional issues. Having a chronic illness has an adverse effect on your heart and mind. Anxiety, depression, and stress are all present. Guess what, though? Acupuncture is skilled at handling those bothersome guests. It's like having a one-way ticket to paradise from this Zen master, encouraging calmness and telling those stress chemicals to go hiking. It is the body and mind cooperating like a well-oiled machine.

Allow me to reveal a small secret now. I've seen everything. As a physician and health and wellness consultant for many years, I have witnessed firsthand the numerous miracles acupuncture has performed on my patients. They feel as though they've hit a brick wall when they walk in with their battle wounds from Hepatitis E. However, when acupuncture is included in their treatment regimen, patients begin to experience remarkable progress. My friend, it's like there's light at the end of the tunnel.

However, pay attention. Don't go into it believing that acupuncture would take care of all of your issues. My friend, it's not a replacement for traditional medical care. Consider it the tag team champion, complementing the conventional methods, dietary adjustments, lifestyle modifications, and all that jazz. But be sure to work with a qualified acupuncturist who is knowledgeable about liver issues in particular. They will create a customised treatment plan particularly for you and answer all of your urgent concerns.

Here's the skinny, then. Acupuncture treatments are quite simple. These incredibly thin, sterilised needles are inserted into predetermined body spots, and after that, you just lie back and unwind for a good 20 to 40 minutes. How many and how often are the sessions held? That would depend on the severity of your hepatitis E and how well you handle the medication. It's similar to dancing, my friend, and you need to establish your rhythm.

And just one more thing, too. Your acupuncturist may include a few extra treats. A comprehensive regimen including dietary adjustments, lifestyle modifications, and herbal medicine is intended to give your body an extra boost. My friend, it's like a team effort where everyone helps your body's innate healing capabilities so you may take charge of your own health path.

To put it briefly, acupuncture is the best treatment for Hepatitis E. It goes beyond simply increasing liver function and igniting your body's natural healing process. It's about empowering you to shine on the inside and out, mentally and physically. So, my buddy, get aboard the acupuncture bandwagon. Embrace holistic healing, unleash the magic, and conquer your Hepatitis E adventure like a pro. I have faith that you can overcome this.

Herbal Remedies: Nature's Healing Power

You know, there is no history of therapeutic cures that surpasses that of herbal remedies. Really, these things were well known to ancient civilizations, who used plants' medicinal properties to cure a wide range of illnesses. And you know what? Herbal medicines are legitimate for promoting health and wellness, as our ancestors have believed. Modern science is finally catching up and verifying this.

Consider the hepatitis E virus. This terrible illness actually affects the liver, interfering with its normal function and leading to a host of other issues. But have no fear, my friends—some herbal heroes are here to save the day and provide your liver with the care it needs to heal.

Milk thistle, or Silybum marianum if you're feeling fancy, is one such hero. This ancient infant is all about empowering the liver and letting those poisons know who's boss. The key ingredient in milk thistle, silymarin, does wonders in lowering inflammation in the liver and shielding those priceless liver cells from the harm that the hepatitis E virus can inflict.

Let's now discuss turmeric. This spice's ability to reduce inflammation has been gaining attention, and it really works. The primary active ingredient in turmeric, curcumin, offers so many health advantages that it's difficult to list them all. However, its liver-protective properties are what intrigue us, particularly its ability to lessen oxidative stress and inflammation, two factors that are known to increase in the livers of people with hepatitis E. Turmeric is a welcome addition to any Hepatitis E care regimen, whether you take it as a supplement or sprinkle it on your diet.

But there's still more! Ginger, licorice root, schisandra, and dandelion root are all on the same level as the superheroes who like liver. Licorice root has long been used as an Ayurvedic treatment for liver problems; ginger is a powerful anti-inflammatory that can help with detoxification and reduce liver inflammation; dandelion root has long been used to keep livers happy and healthy; and schisandra is a fancy Chinese berry that can detox and protect the liver like nobody's business.

However, while herbal medicines are fantastic, conventional medical care should also be provided in addition to them. Consider them more of your regular treatment's auxiliary personnel, cooperating for the common good. Therefore, before entering the herbal realm, be sure to consult a healthcare professional.

Here's where it gets very cool. You're taking a comprehensive approach to curing Hepatitis E when you include these herbal miracles in your treatment regimen. Addressing the underlying reasons is just as important as treating the outward symptoms. Herbal medicine can therefore support your liver and help you feel better overall, especially when combined with dietary and lifestyle modifications.

Oh, and one more thing: if you don't know what you're doing, the herbal world may be a bit of a jungle. Thus, it's critical to purchase your herbs from reputable vendors and consult an experienced herbalist or healthcare professional. They will provide you with the appropriate herbs and dosages based on your condition and demands.

The beauty of nature is just astounding. She has bestowed upon us an abundance of medicinal benefits, with every herb possessing distinct abilities, particularly concerning liver well-being. So visit nature's pharmacy and accept the wisdom of herbal medicine. You'll soon be surfing the wave to greater health and your liver will thank you for it.

The Mind-Body Connection: Harnessing Your Inner Healing Power

You know, we've always recognised how powerful the mind-body connection is in the field of holistic healing. It's like this age-old knowledge that healers and sages have handed down through the years. They understood long ago that our mental and emotional states might have a significant influence on our physical well-being. And what's this? These days, science fully supports that. Babe, it's all about how our bodies and thoughts interact so intricately. Really, it's intriguing stuff.

So, take this. Research has indicated that long-term stress, depressive feelings, and a pessimistic view of life can seriously impair our health. Our bodies create a lot of stress hormones, such as cortisol, when we're anxious or depressed, and these hormones might compromise our immune system. Do you understand what that implies? We are more vulnerable to many different illnesses, such as Hepatitis E. Must be nuts, huh?

On the other hand, developing an optimistic outlook, finding methods to decompress, and engaging in joyful activities? Man, that really can change everything. It really is like having a secret weapon for treating hepatitis E. And one technique that has recently gained a lot of popularity is meditation. We can all access this inner healing force by clearing our minds and living in the present. Like, actual studies have demonstrated that regular meditation can improve our immune systems, lower blood pressure, and help us cope with stress. In all honesty, it's a huge game-changer for Hepatitis E management.

What else is really awesome? Visualization. It all boils down to vividly picturing good and healthful consequences in your mind. When we visualise ourselves as lively, disease-free, and well, we are sending strong signals to our subconscious mind, which in turn impacts our actual body. And you know what? Studies have indicated that visualisation has the potential to improve immune response and trigger the body's own healing processes. It is very genuine, yet it feels magical.

Also, are you familiar with deep breathing? It's one of those mind-body connection tools that is both easy and effective. This component of our neural system that promotes relaxation is activated when we take deep breaths, such as those belly breaths. You won't believe it, but deep breathing gives our blood more oxygen and soothes our thoughts. It's as if our entire body receives a reset, assisting our innate healing mechanisms. I think that's quite remarkable.

To be honest though, adopting a positive outlook is among the most crucial things we can do to manage hepatitis E. It is, after all, quite normal to experience fear or frustration when managing a chronic condition. But it won't help us to cling to those unfavourable feelings. Nope. We cultivate this space inside of ourselves that promotes healing and resilience by consciously choosing to concentrate on thankfulness, optimism, and positive thinking. It seems as though we're preparing our bodies to kick Hepatitis E in the ass.

And believe me when I say that self-care is vital to the whole mind-body connection game. engaging in enjoyable activities, such as exploring the outdoors, taking up a hobby, and spending time with close friends and family? Babe, that's not simply a luxury. When it comes to controlling a chronic illness such as Hepatitis E, it is an absolute must. You know, we need to take care of ourselves.

Now, in addition to all of the exercises we've covered, there are other supplementary methods that have the potential to greatly enhance the mind-body connection. I'm referring to practises such as energy healing, massage therapy, acupuncture, acupressure, and herbal medicine. All of them focus on restoring equilibrium to our body's energy systems and igniting our innate healing processes. It feels as though we are maximising our general well-being and health. That's really cool.

But what's the deal? When it comes to controlling Hepatitis E, coping mechanisms are key. Finding good coping mechanisms for stress and hardship is crucial when navigating the difficulties of a chronic illness. Do you have any idea how those tactics would appear? Perhaps it's talking to our loved ones for support, going to therapy or support groups, learning stress-reduction strategies, or even just finding creative ways to express ourselves. We may lessen the effects of stress on our bodies and improve our chances of healing by developing our inner fortitude and resilience.

See, this notion of a mind-body connection? It has enormous power. It's as though we always have this hidden tool in our back pockets to aid with our bodies' innate healing abilities. We can improve our general welfare and effectively manage Hepatitis E by adopting coping mechanisms, using relaxation techniques, and maintaining an optimistic outlook. But, as they say, each person's journey is unique. Hence, the key is to experiment with several approaches and determine which ones work best for us. We will delve even further into diet, exercise, and lifestyle modifications in the upcoming chapter. We'll provide you with some doable tips for controlling your Hepatitis E while leading a fantastic life. Remember that you can handle this, sweetie. No matter what obstacles you encounter, you possess the ability to succeed. I'm confident that you will lead a vibrant life.

The Role of Nutritional Therapy in Hepatitis E Management

Let me tell you, it's not easy to manage hepatitis e. A thousand balls to juggle at once is how it feels. The point is, though, there are a number of approaches you may take to treatment; one of them is nutritional therapy; believe me, this will completely transform your condition.

Imagine this: during Hepatitis E, your liver, the unsung hero that cleans your blood of all impurities, requires a little additional care. Thankfully, nutritional treatment can help with that, my buddy. It all comes down to providing your liver with the proper nutrition so that it can recover and perform at its peak.

I mean, load up your plate with foods high in antioxidants. These bad boys are like an army battling off free radicals, which have the potential to really harm your liver. Consider colourful fruits like juicy berries, leafy greens that tantalise the senses, and bell peppers that give your meals a rush of flavour. By adding these superfoods to your diet, you're providing your liver with the defence it requires.

That's not all, though. We must also discuss the powerful omega-3 fatty acids. These offspring can be found in nuts and seeds, as well as fatty seafood like mackerel and salmon. They are incredibly effective in lowering inflammation, which is something you most definitely don't need more of when you have Hepatitis E. So stock up on these good fats and let them to do their magic on your physique.

Not to mention the importance of protein. This nutrient is essential to the game of liver health. It functions similarly to the key component your liver need for detoxification. Here, we're talking about lean protein sources like turkey, chicken, and lentils. They will assist in healing those cells in addition to supporting your liver.

Hey, it's not all about the specific nutrients. It also has to do with the wider picture. The key is to follow a diet high in whole foods. Fill up on crisp vegetables, lean proteins, substantial whole grains, and fresh fruits. Your liver will receive all the nutrients it needs from these treats. Additionally, avoid such processed foods at all costs because they are loaded with harmful ingredients and fats. Rather, choose complete, high-nutrient foods because that's where the actual magic is found.

Let's now discuss hydration. When it comes to nutritional therapy for Hepatitis E, this is significant. It is imperative that you maintain adequate hydration, since it truly does. Here, water is your greatest ally. Continue to sip it throughout the day. Additionally, please minimise your intake of alcoholic or sugary drinks. I promise you that they're not doing your liver any favours.

But hold on, we're not quite finished. Let's discuss lifestyle instead than just eating. Now is the moment to move. Frequent exercise is essential. It increases your liver's sensitivity to insulin, which is very beneficial. Additionally, it increases blood flow, lowers inflammation, and promotes heart health. Choose an activity regimen that suits you best, whether it be strength training or aerobic, and watch your liver grow.

Not to be overlooked is tension. It can cause severe damage to your health, particularly if you have a persistent ailment such as Hepatitis E. Techniques for stress management are therefore equally crucial. Try some yoga, deep breathing, or mindfulness meditation. Discover your inner peace and allow it to heal your liver and improve your general health.

Finally, but just as importantly, look after your emotional and mental well-being. It can be difficult to live with Hepatitis E, and it's okay to experience a range of emotions. Seek expert assistance if necessary. Using psychology-related strategies and counselling can significantly improve the way that emotional distress, anxiety, and depression are managed. The most important thing in this situation is to look after yourself, my friend.

There you have it, then. The undiscovered weapon in the fight against Hepatitis E is nutritional therapy. A balanced diet rich in antioxidants and omega-3 fatty acids can support liver function and improve general health. Make those small dietary adjustments and lifestyle improvements, and observe the transformation of your body. My buddy, food truly is medicine, and you never know where this path can take you—into a better, healthier life.

Exploring Traditional Chinese Medicine

Now, let me explain about hepatitis E. Do you realise that the main goals of traditional medicine are to support the liver and alleviate symptoms? Traditional Chinese Medicine (TCM) employs an alternative methodology. It treats the underlying imbalances that cause the ailment in the first place and takes a holistic approach to treating the body. TCM recognises that Hepatitis E is a manifestation of an imbalance throughout your body, not just an illness of the liver.

This idea of Qi is central to TCM. Think of it as the force that sustains your life. It moves through the meridians, which are these energy channels in your body. You're healthy when everything is in balance and in motion. However, you can become ill if there is an obstruction or imbalance in the flow of Qi. According to TCM, hepatitis E is caused by a disruption in the Qi flow of the liver, which results in inflammation and malfunction.

TCM has several tricks up its sleeve to help you heal and bring your Qi back into balance. They make use of acupuncture, herbal remedies, and even nutritional therapy. First, let's talk about herbal formulas. TCM doctors recommend particular mixes of herbs and minerals to address various parts of the illness. It's similar to a specially made cocktail for your particular situation.

TCM herbal remedies for Hepatitis E concentrate on strengthening your immune system, decreasing inflammation, and enhancing your liver. Researchers have discovered that certain herbs, such as schisandra, milk thistle, and pleurum, can shield your liver from hepatitis E-related damage. These herbs aid in your body's healing process because of their potent anti-inflammatory and antioxidant qualities.

But there's still more. Acupuncture! This is the procedure when very tiny needles are inserted into designated acupuncture spots on your body. These sites can affect your Qi flow and are connected to several organs. TCM practitioners can help you feel better overall and restore liver equilibrium by focusing on certain acupuncture points.

Studies have indicated that in Hepatitis E patients, acupuncture can really lessen viral replication and enhance liver function. It also relieves symptoms like nausea, exhaustion, and even that bothersome stomach ache. It's akin to a rejuvenating physical and mental experience, improving your ability to manage all the negative aspects associated with having Hepatitis E.

Now, the diagnosis methods employed by TCM differ slightly from your own. They use observation, palpation, and a litany of questions to determine the state of your body. To get a sense of what's going on inside of you, they will examine your skin, feel your pulse, and examine the colour and coating of your tongue. It seems as though they are using their fingers to play detective.

The crucial point is that TCM cannot treat Hepatitis E on its own. You still have to collaborate with your usual medical team and heed their guidance. Traditional Chinese medicine (TCM) is a useful adjunct to conventional medicine. Furthermore, in order to ensure that the therapy you receive is both safe and successful, you should locate a qualified TCM practitioner with experience treating liver issues.

Thus, avoid playing around before consulting your healthcare staff. They can explain to you the possible advantages of TCM as well as any strange interactions that might occur between it and your present course of therapy. You have the best chance of managing Hepatitis E and leading the best possible life when conventional medication and TCM work together.

Briefly put, TCM is really beneficial if you have Hepatitis E. Using acupuncture, herbal remedies, and customised treatment regimens, TCM aims to restore your body's equilibrium and promote internal healing. You can live a longer, healthier life by integrating traditional Chinese medicine with TCM. Just don't forget to be in constant contact with your medical staff. You two can conquer this!

Empowerment Through Education

The Power of Knowledge

It wasn't until I saw the effect that information may have on the treatment of a disease like hepatitis E that I really understood the power of knowledge. One's life can actually be changed by it. I will always remember my patient Anna, who was diagnosed with hepatitis E and came to me feeling confused and overwhelmed. She went online for information, just like most people do, out of concern that there would be too much false information to sort through.

However, destiny had another plan for Anna. She happened into trustworthy sites that provided current and accurate information on Hepatitis E. It was similar to discovering a gold box buried beneath choppy seas. Now that she knew more, Anna felt empowered to take charge of her health.

Anna approached managing her disease head-on, resolving to make major lifestyle adjustments. She became aware of the significance of a healthy diet and began eating items that were good for her liver. She continued after that. Anna discovered the key to consistent exercise and incorporated it into her everyday regimen. But Anna's transformation went beyond her appearance; she also looked for online forums and support networks to connect with people going through comparable experiences. In addition to providing emotional support, these relationships provided insightful advice on navigating the challenging terrain of Hepatitis E.

Through proactive involvement in her own treatment, Anna navigated the intricate world of Hepatitis E. She worked hard with her medical team to create a customised treatment plan that catered to her particular goals and needs. Anna made sure her treatment was successful and long-lasting by scheduling frequent check-ups and maintaining open lines of communication.

Though it's merely the beginning, Anna's narrative is a brilliant example. It demonstrates the critical role that knowledge plays in the management of hepatitis E. People can acquire a true understanding of the virus and how it affects their health by obtaining correct information. They can investigate the various therapy choices and identify any potential dangers or problems.

Empowerment and knowledge have always been my guiding concepts in medicine. I think it's important to give my patients the information they need to make wise decisions regarding their health. I urge them to look for trustworthy sources, pose inquiries, and take an active role in their own care.

Understanding is not limited to treating the physical symptoms of Hepatitis E; it is also essential for mental health. People can face their concerns and anxieties head-on by understanding the infection and all of its implications. They can build ways to deal with the turns and turns that life may throw at them and rely on specialists and loved ones for support.

In the end, the secret to controlling hepatitis E is understanding. People can take an active role in their own care and make educated decisions if they take the time to learn about the virus. They can make lifestyle adjustments including eating better, exercising, and learning stress-reduction techniques. They might also look into alternative and complementary therapies that can provide more assistance.

I therefore want to leave all of my readers with this advice: never undervalue the importance of knowledge in managing hepatitis E. Accept it and allow it to direct you as you go toward total control. Hepatitis E can cause obstacles in life, but with the right combination of medical care, emotional support, lifestyle modifications, and self-care practises, people can live happy, meaningful lives. You have the ability to alter your life; all you need is a desire to learn new things and the courage to choose this life-altering path.

Navigating the Healthcare Maze

I'll tell you what, the healthcare system may be really intimidating. particularly if you're battling an illness like hepatitis E. It's like attempting to find your way through an insane maze, but don't worry. I'm here to offer some advice on how to survive intact because I've been there, done that.

First and foremost, you need to take the initiative. Instead of letting the system overwhelm you, don't just sit there. Learn the ins and outs of your illness and arm yourself with knowledge by educating yourself about it. It really does make a big impact, I promise. Knowing what's happening allows you to take an active role in your own treatment, ask the proper questions, and come to well-informed conclusions. It's similar to taking charge of and directing your own path to better health.

Prepare yourself now, as things are going to become a little complicated. I am aware that the medical language they use will make your head spin. The thing is, though, you have to seize those medical terminology by the horns and take them by force. Learn the vocabulary and concepts related to hepatitis E. Although it may seem like a whole new language to learn, it's essential for efficient communication with your healthcare team. And believe me when I say that being able to comprehend what they're saying and vice versa is revolutionary.

This is where communication is key, my buddy. It all comes down to forming a strong alliance with your healthcare team. Don't hold back or be timid. Talk for a long time without stopping. Put all of your worries, uncertainties, and expectations on the table. You are the best person to know about your body and yourself, even though they are the experts. You can make sure your healthcare providers notice you, hear you, and give you the treatment you really need by taking an active role in your relationship with them.

However, pay attention, my friend—you need to stand up for yourself. I have to emphasise this again. Here, we are discussing your health. And occasionally you have to take a stand and say something. Seek clarification if something is unclear. Never be reluctant to discuss alternate treatment alternatives or to get second views. You will receive the greatest care possible if you use your voice, which matters.

Let's take a moment to consider ideas beyond the realm of medicine. In my experience as a health and wellness coach, combining complementary and alternative methods can have a profound impact. Chronic illnesses such as Hepatitis E can be effectively managed with the use of many interventions, including food planning, lifestyle modifications, counselling, and self-care practises. It's similar to including more components in your treatment plan, improving your general health, and assisting with conventional medical care.

All right, let's get to work. Taking care of your health must be your first concern. And you must maintain thorough records in order to achieve it. I'm referring to all of your medical records, including notes from appointments, test findings, and treatment plans. You're always informed, much like if you had your own personal journal tracking your health journey. It also helps when you need to acquire a second opinion or talk about your health with your medical professionals. It's like having all the tools you need to win the war on healthcare, I promise.

The fact is that you cannot accomplish this on your own. You require a network of allies. Your team, ride or die. Your friends and family can assist with daily chores, accompany you to doctor's visits, and offer emotional support. Hey, don't underestimate the strength of community. Support groups devoted only to Hepatitis E are available. Make connections with those who are experiencing similar circumstances. They can be your lifeline when times are hard since they have insights, understand the hardships, and are understanding.

As the curtain rises on this maze of healthcare, keep the following in mind: be proactive, speak out when necessary, stand up for yourself, think outside the box, preserve your documentation, and rely on your network of support. You have the ability to confidently navigate your health journey, my friend. I promise you, you can succeed.

Building a Support Network

Managing a medical condition such as hepatitis E is like to attempting to navigate a maze while wearing a blindfold. It is like attempting to find a needle in a haystack, there is so much information available. But don't worry, I can help you navigate with these pointers.

Finding reliable information sources should be your top priority. I'm referring to trustworthy research papers, competent healthcare providers, and trustworthy websites. These are the covert tools at your disposal to combat hepatitis E. You can take control of your health and make educated decisions about your treatment options if you have access to correct information.

However, we must not undervalue the importance of connections. Being afflicted with Hepatitis E might make you feel as though you're the only person on a remote island. It's crucial to reach out to those who are experiencing similar circumstances. Online discussion boards and support groups are excellent places to start. You can establish connections with genuine understanding individuals worldwide. It is like to discovering an oasis amidst a desert.

Don't stop there, either. Look for Hepatitis E support groups or local organisations. These people provide a variety of social gatherings, activities, and educational seminars where you can interact with people in person. Developing connections inside your own neighbourhood might be similar to discovering a valuable hidden gem. It provides you with an immediate support network and a feeling of acceptance.

However, we must also consider the emotional aspect of the situation. It can be difficult to manage a chronic condition, and it can negatively impact your mental health. Your friends and family can help with that. Talk to them about your worries, fears, and accomplishments. Give them an opportunity to support you. A listening ear can often be all you need to lighten the weight.

Support groups and counselling, on the other hand, are your best bet if you're searching for a more structured method. Comparable to a life raft in a stormy sea are these resources. They offer a secure space where you may communicate your feelings, pick up coping mechanisms, and get advice from knowledgeable experts. It can change everything to speak with someone who is aware of the emotional torment associated with hepatitis E.

Let's now discuss receiving assistance from the most significant individual in your life: you. This is the time to practise self-care. It all comes down to making the time to care for your body, mind, and spirit. To maintain your inner serenity, engage in mindfulness and meditation. Take up activities that calm and make you happy. Remember to give your physical well-being first priority by getting regular exercise and eating a balanced diet. By taking care of yourself, you're laying a solid foundation for overcoming Hepatitis E's obstacles.

In summary, developing a robust support system is your covert tool in the fight against hepatitis E. It's about obtaining trustworthy information, making connections with like-minded people, asking family and friends for emotional support, and looking out for your own wellbeing. Recall that you are not travelling this path by yourself. There are people and resources available to support you. Notwithstanding the challenges that you face, you possess the ability to take charge of your well-being and lead a satisfying life. So let's get ready and take on Hepatitis E.

Unleashing Your Inner Advocate

Receiving a Hepatitis E diagnosis might be like having a tonne of bricks fall on you. It's this overwhelming sense of not knowing, as if you're lost in a huge maze and have no map. The problem is, though, that you are in charge of this bizarre path towards better health. My friend, you are in charge. And I'm here to teach you how to find your inner champion and handle this crazy world of managing hepatitis E with confidence.

Prioritize your education first. Being well-informed is crucial when it comes to your health since "knowledge is power." Explore the world of hepatitis E in great detail. Find more about the possible side effects, causes, symptoms, and remedies. Become well-informed so that you may engage in meaningful dialogue with your healthcare team. But keep in mind that you should only believe credible sources, such as medical websites and expert advice. Avoid those dubious sources that can make you feel even more puzzled.

Next, assemble a strong support system around yourself. With Hepatitis E, you don't have to fight it alone. Speak with your friends, family, and medical professionals; they can offer you the emotional support, direction, and inspiration you require. And don't overlook those in-person and virtual support groups. These people have been there before, so they can provide unique perspectives and counsel that you won't find anywhere else. I promise you, their assistance will be your lifeline.

Let's now discuss how to communicate effectively with your healthcare team. When it comes to controlling your hepatitis E, these people are the real deal. Thus, it's imperative that you have open and transparent channels of contact with them. Make a list of your questions, concerns, and any changes to your condition or symptoms before your appointments. Engage in active participation in the discussions at those appointments. Never hesitate to voice your views and concerns or to seek for clarification. Make sure you have a voice in the decisions that are made because you are on this journey together.

Let's dive right in and learn about insurance coverage. Keeping Hepatitis E under control can be an expensive journey, so it's critical to understand what your insurance policy includes. Learn about the specifics. Does your plan provide coverage for lab tests, doctor visits, prescription drugs, and hepatitis E-related procedures? Do not give up if you have any difficulties with insurance. For further information, get in touch with your insurance company; better yet, ask a patient advocate or medical billing specialist for help. They'll look out for you.

You may be apprehensive about this next bit, but bear with me: taking part in research studies and clinical trials. I realise that this sounds like we're going somewhere unknown. The truth is that these experiments and trials are advancing medical understanding and leading to the creation of novel therapies. You become a superhero for the scientific community as well as for yourself by taking part. You may even be able to receive state-of-the-art medical care. Just remember to have a candid discussion about the advantages and disadvantages with your medical staff.

Now, my buddy, get comfortable as we discuss developing self-advocacy abilities. This is the point of personalization. It all comes down to hone your forceful communication abilities and conducting independent research on available treatments. Never hesitate to get second opinions when necessary. Here, it's you who makes the decisions. Maintain a record of your symptoms and development, and speak up for yourself so that you can get the assistance and care you need. After all, you are the star of this show.

Let's now concentrate on lifestyle adjustments. Hepatitis E is a difficult condition, but by adjusting your daily routine, you can lessen some of the discomfort. Think about implementing a nutritious diet, exercising frequently, practising yoga or meditation to reduce stress, and obtaining a good night's sleep. And remember to discuss with your healthcare staff any specific dietary or lifestyle adjustments that may be helpful. Maintaining your general health will help you on your path to overcoming hepatitis E.

The mental and emotional toll that Hepatitis E causes is something we cannot overlook. It wears me out, buddy. Therefore, getting mental and emotional assistance is essential. It's acceptable to get in touch with a counsellor or therapist who focuses on chronic illness. They will rescue you from the choppy waves of this illness, acting as your emotional lifeguard. Remember such support groups as well. Being in the company of people who genuinely get what you've been through can alter everything. And who knows? You might find comfort in journaling, practising mindfulness, or engaging in activities that truly ignite your soul. You merit that burst of happiness.

Lastly, let us not overlook your contribution to spreading awareness of Hepatitis E as you embrace your inner champion. Keep up with the most recent findings, available treatments, and modifications to policy. Participate in awareness campaigns and spread the word about your experience. Knowledge is strength, my companion. Additionally, by raising awareness of Hepatitis E, you're helping individuals who are affected by it have a better future.

It's not simple to let your inner advocate out. My friend, the war is still ongoing. But as you move forward, you're equipping yourself with the skills and information necessary to respond. Get informed, establish a support system, express your demands, comprehend your insurance, engage in research, develop your capacity for self-advocacy, consider changing your way of life, receive emotional support, and raise the awareness bar. You can do this. You underestimate your strength. Let's defeat hepatitis E together.

Educating Others: Spreading Awareness

You know, effective communication is really vital when it comes to increasing awareness about Hepatitis E. We need to make those facts widely known in a manner that is clear to all. Simple language that is understandable to all is used instead of technical medical phrases or complex jargon. We do not wish to overburden those who are not medical specialists, you know?

But my friend, it's not simply about providing the facts. We must likewise aggressively dispel those bothersome falsehoods and misconceptions. I tell you what, spreading false information can result in severe discrimination and stigma. And for those with Hepatitis E, that is the very last thing we want. Let's debunk those rumours by presenting correct information and correcting the record.

This is when the real fun starts: advocacy. Yes, what I said was accurate. We need to push for laws and programmes that aid in diagnosis, treatment, and prevention. This include encouraging immunizations, advocating for increased financing for research and novel therapies, and educating the public about safe measures to stop the disease from spreading.

But who will emerge from this drama as the victor? Why, with me, my friend, and you. We can encourage people to take initiative and effect positive change by imparting our knowledge and experiences. There are a plethora of options for achieving this goal, including coordinating educational workshops, planning awareness campaigns, or forming alliances with nearby healthcare facilities and community organisations. Man, we have to be the cause's ambassadors.

Now, wait a moment. Remembering that every audience is unique is crucial. Certain people may require information based on their age, culture, or educational attainment. We have to get to every one of them. To spread the word to as many people as we can, let's employ every resource at our disposal, including social media, websites, brochures, and community activities.

The important thing to remember is that we need to talk to people, buddy. Interact with them. Hold talks, organise seminars, and get people together for get-togethers in the neighbourhood. People should feel free to ask questions and look for information in a safe area that we need to establish. We need to allay their fears and worries around Hepatitis E.

Well, there's still more. Learning never stops. It is imperative that we be informed about the recent advancements in the field of hepatitis E. Participate in online forums, read all those scholarly papers, and attend conferences. By remaining knowledgeable, we may give others trustworthy and correct information, which can truly help.

The true hidden weapon, however, is right here: storytelling. Yes, what I said was accurate. It changes everything when people with Hepatitis E share their own experiences. You won't believe the emotional connection it makes and the empathy it fosters in others. It really hits home when we hear about those firsthand accounts. It serves as a timely reminder of the significance of early diagnosis, prevention, and treatment. Furthermore, it motivates people to take up initiatives in their own communities and lives.

It's obvious as day, my friend. The key to our collective survival is raising awareness about hepatitis E and educating others about it. Making a genuine difference occurs when we engage with people, dispel myths, fight for change, become ambassadors, adapt our message, communicate clearly, never stop learning, and share our experiences. Let's build a future in which Hepatitis E is only a fading memory.

Overcoming Stigma

Unmasking the Hidden Pain

Let me introduce you to Sarah. She's this young, ambitious, passionate woman with a lot of goals. But when she was afflicted with hepatitis E in her undergraduate years, life threw her a curveball. I can see this mixture of vulnerability and sadness in Sarah's eyes now when she talks about her trip. When she learned of her diagnosis, it was as if everything in her world had collapsed, destroying her hopes and dreams. And it continued after that. She felt so very alone since the stigma and the fear of being judged became her regular companions.

The day Sarah made the decision to tell a close friend about her health is one that she will never forget. She was sorely mistaken in her assumption that she would find sympathy and understanding. Instead, terrified of contracting the infection and bearing the stigma, her buddy became frightened and withdrew from society. Just picture how Sarah felt about that. It felt like a blow to the core of her being. She was rejected by someone she trusted, and the emotional devastation that followed was indescribable.

The unfortunate thing is that Sarah's tale is not special. Similar discrimination and rejection are experienced by a great number of patients with Hepatitis E when they disclose their condition. It's as like there's an unseen anguish that pierces their spirits deeply, damaging their emotional stability and sense of self.

I began to understand that this concealed suffering touched every part of their lives as I continued to go deeper into my studies and speak with more people. Their anxiety and depression become their daily companions, carrying the weight of stigma with them all the time. They begin to doubt their value and position in society, experiencing a sense of alienation.

Consider Jacob as an example. He distanced himself from everyone and everything because of hepatitis E. If people found out about his condition, he was afraid of the assumptions and judgement that would ensue. He withdrew from social interactions as a result, imprisoning himself in solitude. The way this concealed grief gradually undermines their self-esteem and causes them to feel so cut off from the outside world is sad.

Having Hepatitis E implies that you must always carry the stigma with you. It's like concealing this enormous weight inside while putting on a veneer of normalcy. They hide their sickness out of fear of being rejected, which keeps them from getting the help they sorely need.

But we can no longer allow this secret suffering to be unseen. We must bring it to light. We can better comprehend these courageous people's hardships by hearing their personal stories. The terrible effects that stigma has on people's mental and emotional health must be acknowledged. It's time to end the taboo and establish a compassionate and healing environment.

I'll go into the coping mechanisms and self-help approaches that Hepatitis E patients have found useful in addressing this pain that is hidden in plain sight in the next section. We will also discuss the significance of self-acceptance, support systems, and ending the stigmatisation loop. It all comes down to giving these people the confidence to accept who they really are and dispel the myths about their illness. By working together, we can create a society that is inclusive, understanding, and compassionate.

Yes, even if the invisible suffering that many with hepatitis E carry doesn't have to remain that way. Let's build a society where compassion and understanding triumph over prejudice and condemnation. It all begins with revealing this concealed suffering and accepting the tales that surround it.

Breaking the Shackles of Shame

Hurt, dude. It is lethal. It really has the power to seize hold of you like a vice, ruining your sense of value and interfering with all aspects of your life. Furthermore, if you have Hepatitis E, the stigma and condemnation you face from society simply makes the burden you already bear much heavier.

Realizing how destructive shame is is the first step towards overcoming it. It's the ingrained conviction that your illness makes you inferior and defective in some way. And believe me when I say that this belief can seriously undermine your self-worth. You begin to feel alone in this mess and guilty and embarrassed.

The problem is that society has a terrible attitude toward hepatitis E. Individuals make a tonne of assumptions and utter absurdities about it. Simply because you have this illness, others perceive you as being unclean or careless. And believe me when I say that—that just heaps on additional guilt.

Your entire life may be ruined by that guilt. Your relationships, employment opportunities, and general quality of life are all negatively impacted. You begin to withdraw from society and isolate yourself out of fear of being looked down upon and rejected. And believe me when I say that—it only serves to heighten the sense of isolation and hopelessness.

But, my friend, here's the thing. You have to realise that shame is really a social construct. It's not an accurate representation of your value or identity. It is something that can be faced with and conquered. All you have to do is regain your self-worth and faith in yourself.

And allow me to present Sarah to you as proof of it. This woman is definitely not to be taken lightly. She has Hepatitis E, and at first she felt like shame had taken over her. Because she believed that her illness would cause her to be condemned eternally, she withdrew and allowed her humiliation to consume her. She then connected with a health and wellness coach, who assisted her in overcoming those self-defeating ideas and realising her own value.

Sarah discovered that her hepatitis E didn't define her after receiving therapy and engaging in significant self-care. She was worthy of love and affection, and her worth extended beyond her physical state. She then began telling her tale, spreading awareness of Hepatitis E, and demonstrating to the world that she wasn't limited by a ridiculous stigma. Others were inspired by her bravery and came to understand that they too could achieve freedom.

And David is the other one. This guy had endured years of living with hepatic encephalopathy and all the associated stigma. He often felt inadequate and compared himself to others who were in good health. He felt that no one would ever accept him for who he was and that his disease rendered him useless.

David, however, later came across a health and wellness coach who assisted him in overcoming those negative ideas. He began to focus on his strengths and changed his attitude through therapy and some serious self-help. He came to see that his experiences had given him an inner strength and special sensitivity that he could utilise to motivate others.

David started promoting knowledge and comprehension of Hepatitis E after gaining more self-assurance. He initiated awareness campaigns, set up support groups, and turned into a ray of hope for other people dealing with the illness. He was not going to allow shame to define him any longer. He regained his worth and took charge of his life.

Now, I'm not saying it's simple to get over shame. Not in a manner. It requires a variety of factors, including a strong support network, expert advice, and a great deal of self-compassion. Most significant, though, is realising that having Hepatitis E does not define you. You have the ability to write your own tale and are valuable just the way you are.

Now, my friend, let's overcome the guilt. Let's accept our value and overcome the criticism of society. We may find the courage to rewrite our own stories and build an empowered community by taking inspiration from these inspiring tales. Let's choose advocacy, self-care, and self-acceptance. Let's take control of our life and demonstrate to the outside world that we will not let any silly label to define us.

For everyone who is drowning in humiliation, I hope this brief anecdote offers as a ray of hope. It's time to live life on our terms, to accept our value, and to be proud of who we are. So, my friend, let's get started. Let's fly by releasing those restraints.

Embracing Vulnerability

Alright, allow me to share with you something. I used to believe that being vulnerable was a sign of weakness and that it should be avoided at all costs. Who wants to be vulnerable and run the danger of being disapproved of or evaluated, after all? However, I can tell you that one of the greatest life-changing things we can do for ourselves is to embrace vulnerability. It provides access to a completely new realm of sincere connections, psychological recovery, and a genuine sense of community. And, hey, I'd love to help you learn Hepatitis E management and embrace vulnerability on this trip, if you're game. I promise it's worthwhile.

The truth is that fear of being judged is one of the main obstacles to accepting vulnerability. It's normal to be concerned about other people's reactions if they learn about your illness. We fear that the people we love about would stigmatise, label, or perhaps ignore us. And what's this? I understand that those worries are quite legitimate. The truth is, though, that showing vulnerability does not imply weakness. In actuality, it requires a great deal of bravery and fortitude to be vulnerable and reveal our own selves.

Allow me to introduce you to one of my patients, Sarah. She experienced the intense feelings of guilt and humiliation that are often associated with living with a chronic illness when she was told she had Hepatitis E. She was afraid that her loved ones would judge her and that it would ruin their relationship, so she was afraid to inform them. So what actually transpired? Sarah closed herself off from the outside world because she felt alone and burdened by her illness.

But what's the deal? Sarah eventually plucked up the bravery to tell one of her best friends about her diagnosis. And you know what? Her companion gave a sympathetic and perceptive response. Is it really true? That day, Sarah discovered something really important:

genuine connections can be forged through vulnerability. Because she was no longer concealing this significant aspect of herself, it enabled her to strengthen her relationships. And that voyage she undertook? Well, it gave her the confidence to ask for the help she needed and to open up to others. It guided her toward resilience and emotional recovery. Very amazing, isn't that right?

To be honest with you, it's not easy to disclose our Hepatitis E status. It's difficult, emotional, and demands our vulnerability. I, however, have your back. Would you mind if I shared some useful tactics with you to help ease this whole vulnerability thing?

Find yourself a support system first. Find one or two persons in your life that you can confide in and who you feel comfortable telling about your diagnosis. It might be a relative, acquaintance, or even a support group created especially for people with hepatitis E. These folks will support you, listening to your anxieties and fears while also acknowledging and appreciating your accomplishments. You'll get a sense of acceptance from them.

Educate people next. There are many people who are ignorant about Hepatitis E, and this ignorance can result in stigma and misconceptions. Thus, it is your responsibility to teach those you love. Provide them with information, direct them to available resources, and remain available to address any queries they may have. This will allay their worries and provide room for talks that are empathetic.

Remember to acquire expert assistance as well. See a counsellor or therapist who specialises in managing chronic illnesses like Hepatitis E. Since they are the specialists, they can provide you with direction, emotional support, and coping mechanisms that are specific to your requirements. When it comes to managing the emotional rollercoaster that accompanies having a chronic illness, therapy is revolutionary.

Lastly but not least, practise self-compassion. It can be quite frightening to embrace vulnerability, yet it's acceptable to experience fear, anxiety, or uncertainty. Permit yourself to feel those things, and remind yourself that being vulnerable is a brave thing to do rather than a sign of weakness. Treat yourself with kindness while you go through this.

I can assure you that by embracing vulnerability, you will not only find strength in telling your storey, but you will also build networks and support systems that will be very helpful to you while you manage your Hepatitis E. Thus, keep in mind that vulnerability is not something you have to bear by yourself. In actuality, it's a chance for development, recovery, and acceptance.

The Healing Power of Compassion

I have to share with you this amazing tale of Sarah, this case study if you will, about this amazing woman. Sarah is diagnosed with hepatitis E, is that correct? How hard must that have impacted her, you can only imagine? She felt confusion and fear engulf her like a heavy blanket. And the stigma attached to the illness, man? She felt alone in this struggle and estranged from her loved ones as a result.

But, my friends, here's the thing. Sarah's recovery storey is remarkable, and it all began with kindness. You know, it's like there was some sort of supernatural power that caused her to change? And from whence did it originate? Her wonderful mother, Lisa.

Lisa became a formidable force as soon as Sarah received her diagnosis. Her goal was to become well-versed in all aspects of hepatitis E. She was present at meetings, workshops, support groups, you name it. And believe me when I say that with her newfound wisdom, Lisa transformed into a hero in Sarah's eyes. Not simply a mother, but a ferocious defender of her welfare. She was the family's pillar of support, strong and unwavering.

Oh, and Sarah and Lisa had these in-depth, open discussions about everything pertaining to Hepatitis E, not just the weather. The difficult topics, such as available treatments and emotional challenges, weren't avoided by them. Nope, they took it on together, head-on. Through these exchanges, Sarah came to understand the value of empathy. She could utilise her own storey to combat stigma, spread awareness, and demonstrate to the world that she is more than just a diagnosis.

And let me to introduce you to Sarah's primary care physician, Dr. Patel. That man? He left them speechless. Dr. Patel's focus extended beyond medicine. No, he actually gave Sarah his full attention. He was consoling and guiding her every step of the way, like a personal cheerleader. Sarah genuinely thought she had found the right doctor.

However, Sarah's mother and her physician weren't the only ones who offered support. Even her friends, who at first found it difficult to comprehend her predicament, eventually warmed up. Their viewpoint was altered when they witnessed the compassion and love that her loved ones were exuding. They became informed, attended Sarah's visits, and even planned events to raise money for research on hepatitis E. What a network of support system, huh?

Let me tell you the truth now. It wasn't an easy path for Sarah. There were undoubtedly setbacks. But that kindness, man? It propelled her ahead. She became an advocate for those in similar situations as a result. She reached out to people, shared her experience, and gave them a glimpse of hope. It was like a fire inside of her that found purpose.

And you know what? It's not just Sarah who has compassion. All throughout the world, this amazing power is transforming lives. Hepatitis E patients are truly experiencing life-changing effects. My friends, the power of compassion! It's dismantling the barriers of stigma, encouraging mental health, and fostering an environment where individuals feel understood and supported.

According to all of this studies, compassion is a panacea. Our bodies release the hormone oxytocin when we feel compassion. We feel attached and trusting because of the feel-good stuff. And that really is a game-changer, believe me. decreased stress, enhanced heart health, and a general feeling of wellbeing. It's what who wouldn't want?

But there's still more! My friends, compassion also makes our connections stronger. We become extremely sensitive to the pain of others when we engage in self-compassion practises. We reply with compassion and goodwill. And whoa! Our communities turn into safe havens, and our relationships with our loved ones get closer.

And the best part is right here. It's not just about me or you, compassion. It's the effect of ripples. Compassionate behaviour has a cascading effect of acceptance and understanding on others. One act of kindness at a time, we can destroy the stigma. By sharing tales like Sarah's, we encourage people to develop compassion for themselves.

So allow me to leave you with this, fellow readers. It's not only a passing feeling, is compassion. It's a habit that is deeply ingrained in us. Stories such as Sarah's teach us to be compassionate in our own lives. And by doing this, we set off a chain reaction that, one kind deed at a time, has the power to alter lives and affect the entire planet.

Forging Resilience in the Face of Judgment

Let me tell you, having hepatitis E is like having two swords. On the one hand, you can control it with appropriate medical attention and lifestyle modifications. However, the stigma associated with it can seriously affect one's mental health. You know, people simply don't get it. They treat you unfairly, condemn you, and give you the impression that you are alone on a tiny island. That's hard.

The fact is, though, that we have no responsibility for their lack of comprehension. It's their fault. We must overcome their ignorance and demonstrate to them that we are more than just a medical diagnosis. We are able to handle anything that comes our way because we are strong and resilient. My friend, it's all about perspective.

The secret is self-compassion. We need to practise self-compassion and self-forgiveness when we feel inadequate. Yes, it's simple to feel inferior or ashamed, but we must keep in mind that having hepatitis E does not define who we are. That's not even close to who we are. We fight our fights with courage and grace because we are warriors.

And believe me, everything can be changed by rephrasing those unfavourable sentiments. It's important for us to turn the narrative around and emphasise our strengths when someone calls us unclean or infectious. We take excellent care of our health, and we should be really proud of that. Reject those unfavourable assumptions and rewrite our own narrative.

My friend, the key lies in developing inner strength. It originates from a place deep within—that unshakable faith in our own abilities to overcome any challenge. It is imperative that we tend to our needs, establish limits, and surround ourselves with positive people. We develop the inner power that will see us through the hardest of times in this way.

My friend, I've provided you with some useful tools here. It all comes down to developing an inner strength, rephrasing those unfavourable ideas, and practising self-compassion. You can live your best life and rise above the bullshit if you have these in your toolbox. It takes time to become resilient, but I assure you that with commitment and effort, you can do it.

Now, take what I've given you and transform it into something unique. Recognize your value and your limitless potential. You are not defined by what other people think of you. You are a formidable opponent, my friend. After reading this, I hope you're motivated and prepared to take on anything comes your way. I have faith that you can overcome this.

Thriving With Hepatitis E

The Power of Mindset

I should begin by telling you this bizarre anecdote that really opened my eyes to the true power of mentality. So, I was diagnosed with Hepatitis E a few years ago. It felt like a double gut punch, both mentally and physically. But what's the deal? I chose to approach this issue head-on with a positive perspective there and then, rather of allowing myself to drown in fear and despair.

You see, I genuinely think that our mental states have a significant impact on our physical health. Research supports my claims as well: stress and bad emotions can weaken our immune systems and make it more difficult to fend against diseases. On the other hand, maintaining a cheerful outlook can have a revolutionary effect on our general health and wellbeing.

Therefore, shifting our perspective is the first step towards developing that positive mindset. We may actually use this Hepatitis E situation as a chance for personal development and advancement rather than viewing it as a huge setback or obstacle. I realise this seems insane, but believe me when I say this. We may truly accept our circumstances and take charge of our life if we view them as an opportunity to improve them.

For example, I choose to explore alternate methods of self-care rather than obsessing over how my condition limits me. I began to meditate, practise yoga, and even fully commit to acupuncture. And you know what? These techniques not only made my symptoms better, but they also provided me a wonderful sense of empowerment and control over my health. It's really cool, huh?

Gratitude is a significant component in developing a positive mindset. Dealing with a chronic condition such as Hepatitis E can easily lead to a downward spiral and a forgetfulness of life's positive aspects. However, the reality is that when we consciously choose to be thankful and mindful of our blessings, the tides turn and we are able to recognise the beauty and joy that remain in our lives.

I recall this difficult day when I was experiencing extreme sensations. Rather than stew in annoyance and self-pity, I took out a notepad and wrote down all I had to be grateful for. To just a few, I'm grateful for my supportive friends and family, my family, and the chance to work in the medical industry. That thankfulness moment completely changed my viewpoint and served as a reminder that there is always something positive to be grateful for, even in the worst of circumstances.

Now, cultivating a good outlook also entails gaining a great deal of resilience. It's not easy to manage a chronic condition, let's face it. There will be obstacles in your path, times of annoyance, and a tonne of other stuff. However, if you have a little perseverance, you can overcome all of that and carry on moving forward.

However, resilience is not something we are born with. We can practise and get better at it over time. And practising self-care is one of the finest ways to achieve that. It's true that when we look after our physical, emotional, and mental needs, we strengthen our resilience and maintain an optimistic outlook.

Throughout my experience with Hepatitis E, self-care practises such as journaling, taking regular pauses to refuel, and engaging in pleasant activities have been quite helpful. Not only do these exercises provide me with an energy boost, but they also serve as a reminder of my own perseverance and fortitude. It's akin to a brief motivational speech, you know?

Finally, but just as importantly, I want to emphasise how important it is to ask for help when you need it. It's easy to feel overwhelmed when dealing with a chronic disease, and it can make you feel like the largest outsider. The thing is, though, that magic happens when we connect with others and create a support system.

Seriously. That consolation, inspiration, and useful guidance you receive? It's revolutionary.

Allow me to share a storey with you about a patient of mine who, at a Hepatitis E support group, discovered pure gold. She thought no one could relate to her before she joined, that she was fighting this struggle alone. But my goodness, it was like a quick boost of resilience and optimism when she made connections with people who had been there before. She found a secure place to express her worries and frustrations in the support group, and she also picked up a tonne of helpful hints and techniques for dealing with the condition.

In summary, cultivating an optimistic outlook is crucial for successfully managing Hepatitis E. Changing our viewpoint, being grateful, building resilience, and asking for help are the keys to finding happiness and contentment even in the face of the most difficult obstacles. Thus, let's harness the power of our thoughts to create a promising future. I promise it will be fantastic.

Setting Meaningful Goals

Okay, so let's have a conversation about goal-setting. I understand that having Hepatitis E can present significant difficulties for you, but be aware that this illness does not define you, my buddy. Not in a manner. You have the ability to overcome obstacles and lead a happy life. So let's explore and determine what is really important to you.

Find a comfortable place and think about your priorities. Consider your goals, interests, and ideals. What gives you the feels? What really makes you happy and fulfilled? This self-reflection can help you acquire clarity on your goals and areas of emphasis in this crazy thing we call life, much like a flashlight in the dark.

Now that you have a firm grasp on those priorities, it is time to get to work. And by "business," I mean establishing some clear, attainable objectives that are in line with your genuine priorities. My friend, we're talking about objectives that you can genuinely monitor and achieve. Clearly stated objectives that will help you feel purposeful and directed.

Let's say that wellbeing and self-care are top priorities for you. Excellent decision. My buddy, you matter, and it's crucial that you look after yourself. So let's become modest. Consider adding frequent exercise to your schedule. Perhaps begin with three weekly walks of thirty minutes each. I mean, you're capable of that. The key is to gradually increase your strength and stamina. Little steps, buddy. Any progress is still progress, regardless of its size.

Now that the objectives have been established, let's divide them into manageable chunks. My friend, we're talking about doable measures. Unlock the success road map. Determine the essential behaviours and actions that will help you achieve your objective. Make a timeline after that. What is the frequency of these activities? How long will it last?

Consider the purpose of wellbeing and self-care. Making a schedule for your workouts, choosing an exercise programme that suits you, and monitoring your progress are some examples of your concrete actions. Dissect it, my friend. Keep it in check. We do not wish for you to feel overburdened. You can do this.

Here's where the fun starts: maintaining motivation. It can be difficult to live with Hepatitis E, but don't worry—I've got you covered. It all comes down to figuring out how to maintain that inner fire. Here's a tip that truly works: keep your "why" front and centre. Go inside and recall why it means so much to you to lead a happy and healthy life. Is it for the people you love? To motivate those facing like circumstances? Or perhaps just because you think highly of and are happy with yourself. My friend, put it in writing. Keep your sources of inspiration handy so you can refer to them anytime you need a little pick-me-up.

And by the way, buddy, don't go it alone. Make sure you have a strong support system around you. I am referring to social media platforms, internet forums, or even close friends and family. Seek out others that support and comprehend your trip. You're deserving of that, buddy. Finding a companion with whom to discuss your advancements, difficulties, and successes can have a profound impact.

Let's speak about progress tracking now. It's similar to keeping score, but in a positive sense. To keep track of your progress, pick up a journal, download an elegant app, or do whatever suits you best. Hey, remember to enjoy your victories, no matter how minor they may appear. You're progressing, my friend. You're in command. You're demonstrating to Hepatitis E who is in charge.

But be aware that obstacles will inevitably arise. That's life as it happens, particularly if you have a chronic illness like hepatitis E. But what's the deal? Let those failures not define who you are. Not in a manner. Consider them as chances for development and learning.

If necessary, modify your objectives, but never lose sight of your aspirations or the significance of the journey.

Here's the bottom line, my friend. Establishing those important objectives is similar to having a hidden superpower to survive with hepatitis E. Whatever your challenges, you can create a satisfying and useful life by prioritising your goals, making realistic and detailed goals, breaking them down into manageable steps, maintaining motivation, and monitoring your progress. You possess the fortitude and tenacity to conquer any obstacle in your path. So let's begin this path of self-discovery and goal-setting together and let's demonstrate to the world your true potential. You are a formidable opponent, my friend. Venture forth and prosper.

Discovering Passions and Pursuing Joy

Let me tell you, having Hepatitis E is not easy to live with. It feels like you're always bearing a big burden on your shoulders. It's exhausting on many levels—mentally, emotionally, and physically. The fact is, my buddy, this illness does not have to be the end all be all of our life. It's not the whole damn narrative; it's simply a part of who we are.

Now, if you ask me how to defeat this Hepatitis E beast, I would suggest that the key is to discover what ignites our spirits. My friend, I'm talking about passion. that fierce flame that propels us on under all circumstances. Even when everything else seems to be crumbling, it's that spark that keeps us going.

The first step in discovering our passion is pausing to consider what truly brings us joy. Yes, it's a simple question, but it's difficult to answer. It seems like we've lost sight of what makes us happy because we've been consumed with this illness. I've got your back, so don't worry. I'll lead you through some soul-searching tasks in this chapter to help you rediscover what really excites you.

The truth is that discovering your passion is only the start. The true difficulty is in applying it to our day-to-day activities. I assure you that it is not simple. Our disease requires a great deal of our time and energy. But we can carve out time for our passions with a little preparation and a lot of willpower. I'll share some useful advice with you in this chapter to help you incorporate your passion into your daily activities.

Now, how about we discuss many kinds of passions? The arts provide comfort to some of us. Creative pursuits like writing, painting, or strumming that old guitar in the corner of our room can be lifesaving. They give our feelings a tangible expression by allowing us to spill our emotions onto a canvas or piece of paper. It's also quite therapeutic. So go ahead and experiment with various media and discover your artistic side. You never know when a hidden skill will show itself.

Some of us get our happiness from physical pursuits. Exercise improves both our physical and emotional health, whether we exercise through sports, yoga, or just slaying the dance floor. It improves liver function, reduces stress, and releases feel-good endorphins. Yes, you did hear me correctly. Thus, don't be scared to join in on the fun and get your heart racing. I've got you covered in this chapter, buddy, with advice catered to your specific health requirements.

This, my friend, is the icing on the cake. Do you recall how fulfilling it is to assist others? It's like a eureka moment that makes us stop focusing on our own problems. Giving back to the community gives us a feeling of direction and ties us to something greater than ourselves. Thus, seize the chance to have a positive influence by volunteering or reaching out to people who are facing comparable difficulties. Really, it's a win-win situation.

Let's get one thing clear: being joyful does not entail denying the existence of Hepatitis E or sticking our heads in the sand. No, the key is to not let it to define who we are. It's about proving to ourselves and to the outside world that we are more than a label. We have aspirations, deep desires, and a strong will to experience life to the fullest.

Ultimately, my friend, what enables us to thrive with Hepatitis E is finding our hobbies and pursuing happiness. Reclaiming our life, one day at a time, is the main goal. So grab a seat, and let's set out on this journey of self-discovery where we'll encounter happiness in the most unlikely locations. I assure you, my friend—it will be worthwhile.

Finding Support and Building a Community

I soon learned that only offering medical care wasn't sufficient when I first started my career as a medical doctor and health and wellness consultant. Patients required a complete strategy that addressed their physical, mental, and emotional well-being in addition to medications and prescriptions. That's when it dawned on me: assembling a group of professionals from various wellness and health domains was the best course of action. Our shared objective is to give our Hepatitis E patients the complete treatment and assistance they need, and we strive toward this together.

But when it comes to getting help, where do you even begin? Well, contacting medical experts that specialise in Hepatitis E is one of the first measures. These are the people who can help you with diagnosis, treatment plans, and management techniques because they are knowledgeable and experienced in these areas. They are the ones who can provide you the critical medical attention you require and respond to all of your urgent queries. Therefore, invest some time in building a strong rapport with your healthcare provider—it will be essential to managing Hepatitis E properly.

Let us not overlook the influence that support groups have. These incredible networks unite people who have travelled similar paths, gone through similar experiences, and faced comparable obstacles. And believe me when I say that it may be immensely powerful to be surrounded by people who truly get what you're going through. In addition to finding comfort in company, sharing your experiences, achievements, and worries with other Hepatitis E patients can provide insightful knowledge and coping mechanisms. Support groups provide a secure environment where you may be open and honest without worrying about being judged. And that's priceless, my friend.

Online support communities have seen a sharp increase in popularity in this digital age. For those with Hepatitis E who might not have access to real support groups, these online communities offer a caring setting. Hepatitis E-specific websites and social media platforms can provide you with a plethora of information, resources, and lively discussion threads. Making connections on the internet may be a terrific way to get support and establish a connection with people who genuinely get your path.

However, we must not undervalue the influence of our personal networks. It is vitally important to have a solid support system of friends, family, and loved ones. Even though they might not fully understand all the nuances of Hepatitis E, their understanding and support can be quite beneficial. Inform them of Hepatitis E, be honest with them about your situation, and let them know how they can help. Incorporating your loved ones on your journey fosters a sense of community and shared accountability.

Now, when it comes to support, self-care is something that frequently goes unnoticed. My friend, look after your physical and emotional health. Self-care is crucial, especially while managing a chronic illness like hepatitis E. Take up activities that make you happy and calm, such as hiking, meditation, writing in a notebook, or just being in nature. Make time for the pastimes that bring you joy on a regular basis. Making self-care a priority not only helps you feel better overall, but it also demonstrates to others how to look out for and support you.

Finding support is important, but so is building a network of people who genuinely comprehend and share the difficulties of having hepatitis E. For genuine support and personal progress, it's crucial to surround oneself with people who understand your journey. Thus, don't be afraid to go to conferences, workshops, or events in your community that are related to hepatitis E. These events offer the ideal chance to connect with people who have gone through similar things. Talk to people, hear their tales, and share your own observations. Engaging in community service not only helps the community flourish, but it also helps you make deep connections that feed your spirit.

As a health and wellness coach, I genuinely think that coping mechanisms, alternative and complementary forms of self-care, nutrition and food planning, counselling, psychology, and lifestyle changes have a lot of power. The quality of life for those who have Hepatitis E can be significantly improved by these methods. Since everyone of us follows a different path, I urge you to experiment with these tactics to see which ones suit you the best.

Ultimately, establishing a network and obtaining support are critical to living well with hepatitis E. Remember to join support groups or online forums, ask medical specialists who specialise in treating Hepatitis E for advice, and include your loved ones in your journey. Make self-care a priority and partake in activities that feed every part of your body. Engaging fully in the Hepatitis E community and using holistic methods will help you feel empowered and supported as you go toward recovery. And never forget that you are never alone, my friend—together, we can overcome the obstacles posed by hepatitis E.

Embracing Self-Care and Wellness

I can assure you that living with Hepatitis E is not easy. You feel as though your body is engrossed in an unending tug-of-war, exhausting and overwhelming you. However, remember not to let that depress you. The important thing is to look after yourself, buddy. Managing those symptoms, enhancing your quality of life, and building resilience all come from practising self-care and coping strategies.

Firstly, you need to understand how important it is to prioritise your needs. Hepatitis E is a chronic illness, and managing it can make life extremely hard. Putting self-care first, though, will change your life, I promise. It supports your general well-being and helps you manage your condition better.

In my experience, mindfulness is one method that has changed everything. Indeed, this material is really potent. Being in the moment, judgment-free and detached from past experiences, is the key. Self-awareness and self-compassion are fostered by this profound connection with oneself. Furthermore, I can now manage and comprehend all those feelings and thoughts associated with having Hepatitis E much better thanks to it.

Honestly, my friend, it's not difficult to include mindfulness into your lifestyle. First, dedicate a short period of time each day to concentrating on your breathing. Shut your eyes, find a comfortable place to sit, and take a few deep breaths, allowing the air to fill and exit your body. Without passing judgement, simply acknowledge any ideas or emotions that arise. This easy exercise can improve your general well-being, reduce worry, and quiet the mind.

Now, let us discuss methods for relaxing. It's important to find ways to relax because stress might make your problems worse, dude. Deep breathing techniques, progressive muscular relaxation, visualisation, and guided imagery are all really helpful in my experience. With the use of these strategies, you can relax, reduce heart rate, and feel less tense.

You should be in a calm and serene setting when using these relaxation techniques, dude. Ascertain that no one will break your zen moment by choosing a quiet area free of interruptions. Working through each muscle group in your body, begin by concentrating on your breath. With each exhale, intentionally release any tension. Imagine, for the love of your life, that you are in the most tranquil, pleasing spot to the senses. You'll find that these methods become into superpowers for self-care and a hidden weapon against stress over time.

However, pay attention, my friend—mindfulness and relaxation methods aren't the only things involved. Making decisions that are good for your general health is the key. Exercise, a healthy diet, adequate sleep, and abstaining from drugs and alcohol are all part of that. These lifestyle modifications have the power to boost your body's defences against infection, strengthen your liver, and boost your immune system.

Dude, let's talk about workout. Though it's a pleasant perk, it's not just about appearing strong. Your thoughts and feelings are much improved by regular physical activity. Take part in something you truly enjoy, such as going for a refreshing swim, taking a stroll around the park, or adopting a yoga pose. You will experience an increase in endorphins, a positive mood, and a reduction in the symptoms of anxiety and depression—trust me. Attempt to engage in moderate exercise for at least half an hour on most days, but remember to pay attention to your body's signals and adjust accordingly.

And remember, buddy, moderation is key when it comes to eating. Put your attention on consuming a lot of whole foods—that is, the healthful stuff like fruits, vegetables, whole grains, and lean meats. Man, go ahead and throw away those processed foods, sugar-filled beverages, and saturated fats. Your liver gets the nutrients it needs from a balanced diet, which also maintains your general health.

The ultimate healing magic is sleep, my friend. Every night, try to obtain seven or nine good hours of sleep. Make it a habit to do something relaxing, like take a relaxing bath or read a nice book. A cool, dark, and distraction-free atmosphere is essential for a good night's sleep.

Now for the really good part, buddy. Avoid dangerous chemicals that exacerbate the damage to your liver. Reduce your alcohol consumption or give it up totally. Your liver and alcohol don't mix, my friend. Hey, tobacco, too? It's equivalent to poisoning your liver, dude. So, let's refrain from smoking and breathing in secondhand smoke.

Thus, my friend, you're setting yourself up for success with Hepatitis E by implementing these wellness and self-care routines into your everyday life. Make self-care a non-negotiable component of your strategy and never forget that caring for oneself is not being selfish. It's essential to your health and your capacity to overcome any challenges life may you.

Navigating Relationships and Communication

Relationship-wise, having Hepatitis E may be quite the rollercoaster. I can assure you that it's not an easy task. Managing this situation is similar to wading through a dangerous river, but we can get through it with a little perseverance, comprehension, and effective communication.

The stigma associated with hepatitis E is one of the largest obstacles we face. It resembles being ensnared in an unending web of prejudice and condemnation. It's difficult, I won't lie. We grow lonely and alone because people just don't get it. That's when having a solid support network comes in handy. These people provide consolation, fortitude, and a listening ear when we most need it.

Knowing is power when it comes to relationships. We must inform ourselves and those we care about about hepatitis E. Inform them about its causes, symptoms, and viable treatments. Their misconceptions will vanish once they have the truth, and they will be a rock for us.

But it's also important to communicate our own demands in addition to educate others. With our loved ones, we must be forthright and honest about our limitations and expectations of them. You know, it's like talking to their spirits. If they comprehend our perspective, they will provide us with the assistance we require. However, don't expect them to read minds. It is our responsibility to inform them of our needs.

Conversely, we also need to honour their bounds. Yes, we do require some adjustments from them, but let's avoid adding needless stress. To keep our relationships strong, we need to strike a balance between independence and support.

Not to be overlooked are our healthcare providers. They resemble the primary mentors on this bizarre adventure. We must establish a solid rapport with them, one founded on cooperation and confidence. Seek out an expert on Hepatitis E and pay attention to them. We can ensure that we receive the best care if we actively participate in our healthcare by raising questions and voicing our concerns.

Here's a tip I've picked up recently: prepare ahead of time. Writing down our thoughts helps us communicate effectively with our loved ones and healthcare professionals. Putting our thoughts down on paper helps keep things straight and prevent misunderstandings since sometimes our minds get all mixed up.

Hey, it's not all chatter, though. We must also pay attention. That is, listening intently. We need to demonstrate to our family members and medical professionals that we value their opinions. We must listen to them, endeavour to comprehend them, and ask questions. My friend, it's a two-way street.

And we cannot accomplish this on our own when times are hard. We must look for assistance. Join online or offline support groups to connect with people who are experiencing similar difficulties. It resembles discovering a lifesaver in a raging storm. Those that are exactly like us can provide us with strength, consolation, and affirmation as we share our path with them. These are our stones.

Occasionally, we might need to take things a step further and look for outside assistance. Counselors and therapists can be of great assistance to us in managing our mental health. They have the resources to mentor us, teach us coping mechanisms, and support us as we negotiate the psychological rollercoaster that is Hepatitis E.

Ultimately, the key to living well with hepatitis e is to develop supportive and empowering relationships. We must communicate, set limits, educate, and look for help. Our mental health is just as important as our physical health. And by doing all of this, we may meet the obstacles head-on with grace, resiliency, and unwavering resolve. We can do this.

Celebrating Victories and Milestones

Celebrating successes is an essential aspect of any journey, particularly when coping with a chronic illness such as Hepatitis E. It's simple to become engrossed in the hardships and highs and lows and neglect to stop and acknowledge the victories that have been achieved along the way. But believe me when I say that taking the time to rejoice is what fosters the upbeat and happy environment that drives our advancement and sustains us.

Storytelling is becoming one of our most effective methods for recognising and applauding successes. I mean, when we tell our own tales, we serve as a source of inspiration for others and a constant reminder of our own progress. These tales serve as a kind of monument to our own tenacity and resolve, demonstrating to us that no obstacle is too great to overcome. Every single step we've taken to control our health, from the moment we learned we had a diagnosis, is a win worth celebrating.

One anecdote in particular really resonates with me. It concerns Sarah, a patient who received a Hepatitis E diagnosis two years prior. She was terrified and intimidated by what was ahead when she came to me for the first time. But let me tell you, she handled her symptoms and had an incredibly optimistic attitude on life because to her unyielding drive and the love and support of her family and friends. Sarah is currently living her best life and enjoying each and every victory she achieves in her quest to fully manage her hepatitis E. Whether it's simply being able to go about her everyday activities without feeling worn out or having her liver function back to normal, Sarah's accomplishments are undoubtedly proof of the strength of resiliency.

The truth is that successes can take many different forms. Oftentimes, the smallest, most unimportant moves end up being the greatest victories underground. Making better eating choices, taking our medications as prescribed, or even just finding the will to get up and exercise can all be examples. My friend, those little victories are like the building stones that prepare the way for the greater ones.

Thus, this is what I recommend. In order to truly commemorate these successes, let's establish some significant customs and routines to indicate those benchmarks. It might be as easy as setting aside a short period of time every day to consider our achievements and express thanks for them. Alternatively, we might include our loved ones in our celebration by reaching out to them and allowing them to share in our excitement together. We give our triumphs meaning and purpose when we incorporate these rituals into our life, which makes them even more memorable.

But what's even more awesome? In addition to providing us with the drive and inspiration to keep moving forward, celebrating our successes also helps to strengthen this amazing support system. We become like guiding beacons for anyone who might be having difficulties while enduring their own Hepatitis E journey by sharing our experiences of victory. We provide this environment so that folks can realise they're not fighting this battle alone and can find solace, encouragement, and hope.

And here's the thing to keep in mind: celebrating successes is a continuous practise rather than a one-time event. It goes without saying that there will be challenges and setbacks along the route. But we strengthen this resiliency and unwavering dedication to our own journey by acknowledging and appreciating our successes. When times are hard, we learn to be grateful for the progress we've made and muster the will to keep going.

In conclusion, a crucial component of living well with hepatitis e is acknowledging and appreciating accomplishments. We build this incredible sense of camaraderie and support when we tell one other's stories of tenacity and success, which encourages and drives others to keep going on their own journey to full Hepatitis E control. By engaging in these significant rites and practises, we give thanks for whatever advancement we make, no matter how minor, and give our successes significance and purpose. As we proceed on our path, let's commemorate each and every accomplishment, finding courage and motivation in our individual tales of perseverance. We can continue to grow as a team, my buddy, and encourage others to follow in our footsteps.

Embracing Uncertainty and Finding Resilience

Allow me to delve deeply into the practise of accepting ambiguity and developing fortitude in the face of the unknowable. As a physician and health and wellness coach, I've been there, and I want to share with you my experience as well as useful tips that will help you deal with the unpredictability of Hepatitis E. Believe me, by accepting uncertainty, you can access your inner fortitude and resiliency to overcome every obstacle in your path and not simply survive it.

Uncertainty can be a powerful, terrifying force, but it can also present a chance for development and self-discovery. These uncertain times force us to confront our concerns, reevaluate our convictions, and become flexible. It all comes down to adopting a different perspective, learning to relinquish control, and submitting to the ups and downs of life.

Self-compassion is a crucial component in developing resilience when faced with uncertainty. This is the moment to treat oneself with kindness and gentleness. It's normal to feel a range of emotions, including fear, frustration, grief, and rage, but it's crucial to accept and give meaning to these feelings without passing judgement. You can create a safe space for yourself to process your emotions and find comfort in the face of all the uncertainties by engaging in self-compassion practises.

Mindfulness is another skill for facing ambiguity. It all comes down to living in the present moment to the fullest, free from attachment to the past or the future or judgement. It is possible to notice your thoughts and feelings without becoming overwhelmed by them when you practise inquiry and non-judgment. This helps you gain perspective and clarity by focusing on the things you can control, such as your attitudes, ideas, and behaviours, rather than the things beyond of your control.

Now, while establishing a solid support network is essential for coping with the unpredictability of Hepatitis E, you also need to look after yourself. Discovering activities that feed your body, mind, and spirit is key. Perhaps it entails changing your food, adding exercise to your daily schedule, experimenting with relaxation methods, or learning about complementary therapies like acupuncture or meditation. Making self-care a priority improves your mental and physical health and increases your ability to bounce back from setbacks.

It's important to remember to adjust to change! Your life is significantly altered by hepatitis E, including dietary restrictions, medication schedules, and lifestyle adjustments. But be open to new possibilities and let go of your resistance or resentment towards these developments. Look for other ways to do things, try out new recipes, and get happiness and satisfaction from pursuing new interests and passions. Change can present a chance for development and discovery.

And remember to recognise and rejoice in your little accomplishments along the way as you manoeuvre through the uncertainty. It's simple to become mired in difficulties and disappointments, but it's just as crucial to acknowledge and value each advancement you make, no matter how tiny. Your strength and resolve are demonstrated by every step you take ahead and every instance of resilience. By recognising and appreciating these successes, you foster optimism for the future and a good outlook on life.

It's not easy or comfortable to embrace uncertainty, I won't lie to you. It requires vulnerability, bravery, and a readiness to take a risk. But it's worth it, I promise. By doing this, you can overcome the difficulties of having Hepatitis E by discovering your inner power, resiliency, and potential. Even if the path won't always be easy, you can handle the uncertainty with strength and grace if you have the correct attitude, support network, and self-care routines.

To sum up, uncertainty is a natural element of living well with hepatitis E. It puts your beliefs to the test, forces you to evolve and adapt, and tests your strengths. Through accepting unpredictability and developing resilience, however, you may overcome all those obstacles and not only survive but thrive. It's a journey that calls for perseverance, empathy for oneself, and a steadfast faith in one's own inner power. You can learn to be resilient and have the ability to lead a fulfilling life despite future uncertainties by mastering the skill of embracing uncertainty.Allow me to delve deeply into the practise of accepting ambiguity and developing fortitude in the face of the unknowable. As a physician and health and wellness coach, I've been there, and I want to share with you my experience as well as useful tips that will help you deal with the unpredictability of Hepatitis E. Believe me, by accepting uncertainty, you can access your inner fortitude and resiliency to overcome every obstacle in your path and not simply survive it.

Uncertainty can be a powerful, terrifying force, but it can also present a chance for development and self-discovery. These uncertain times force us to confront our concerns, reevaluate our convictions, and become flexible. It all comes down to adopting a different perspective, learning to relinquish control, and submitting to the ups and downs of life.

Self-compassion is a crucial component in developing resilience when faced with uncertainty. This is the moment to treat oneself with kindness and gentleness. It's normal to feel a range of emotions, including fear, frustration, grief, and rage, but it's crucial to accept and give meaning to these feelings without passing judgement. You can create a safe space for yourself to process your emotions and find comfort in the face of all the uncertainties by engaging in self-compassion practises.

Mindfulness is another skill for facing ambiguity. It all comes down to living in the present moment to the fullest, free from attachment to the past or the future or judgement. It is possible to notice your thoughts and feelings without becoming overwhelmed by them when you practise inquiry and non-judgment. This helps you gain perspective and clarity by focusing on the things you can control, such as your attitudes, ideas, and behaviours, rather than the things beyond of your control.

Now, while establishing a solid support network is essential for coping with the unpredictability of Hepatitis E, you also need to look after yourself. Discovering activities that feed your body, mind, and spirit is key. Perhaps it entails changing your food, adding exercise to your daily schedule, experimenting with relaxation methods, or learning about complementary therapies like acupuncture or meditation. Making self-care a priority improves your mental and physical health and increases your ability to bounce back from setbacks.

It's important to remember to adjust to change! Your life is significantly altered by hepatitis E, including dietary restrictions, medication schedules, and lifestyle adjustments. But be open to new possibilities and let go of your resistance or resentment towards these developments. Look for other ways to do things, try out new recipes, and get happiness and satisfaction from pursuing new interests and passions. Change can present a chance for development and discovery.

And remember to recognise and rejoice in your little accomplishments along the way as you manoeuvre through the uncertainty. It's simple to become mired in difficulties and disappointments, but it's just as crucial to acknowledge and value each advancement you make, no matter how tiny. Your strength and resolve are demonstrated by every step you take ahead and every instance of resilience. By recognising and appreciating these successes, you foster optimism for the future and a good outlook on life.

It's not easy or comfortable to embrace uncertainty, I won't lie to you. It requires vulnerability, bravery, and a readiness to take a risk. But it's worth it, I promise. By doing this, you can overcome the difficulties of having Hepatitis E by discovering your inner power, resiliency, and potential. Even if the path won't always be easy, you can handle the uncertainty with strength and grace if you have the correct attitude, support network, and self-care routines.

To sum up, uncertainty is a natural element of living well with hepatitis E. It puts your beliefs to the test, forces you to evolve and adapt, and tests your strengths. Through accepting unpredictability and developing resilience, however, you may overcome all those obstacles and not only survive but thrive. It's a journey that calls for perseverance, empathy for oneself, and a steadfast faith in one's own inner power. You can learn to be resilient and have the ability to lead a fulfilling life despite future uncertainties by mastering the skill of embracing uncertainty.

Healing From Within

The Healing Journey Begins

Now allow me to take you on a voyage, my friend. a voyage of resilience, learning, and healing. It all began with the initial action I did to begin repairing my body. I knew in my heart that nutrition was the most important factor in my overall health. I therefore assembled a group of specialists, including dieticians and nutritionists, among others. Together, we sat down and designed a customised dietary plan, with an emphasis on items that would promote the health and wellness of my liver.

Vegetables and colourful fruits became my new best pals. Leafy greens, broccoli, cauliflower, and berries. These bad boys helped to detoxify my body and protected my liver from additional damage thanks to their abundance of antioxidants. I was able to recuperate because whole grains like brown rice and quinoa provided me with the essential minerals and energy I needed.

Lean protein intake also gained importance. Beans, salmon, and grilled chicken started to become my go-to protein sources. My liver cells were repaired and rejuvenated by them using their magical touch. Not to mention the importance of healthy fats! Nuts, seeds, and avocados became my tiny assistants, ensuring that my body absorbed all those vitamins and activating my body's defence mechanisms against inflammation.

My friend, it wasn't simply about what I ate. In addition to my medical care, I needed to look into holistic remedies. And oh, did I stumble onto some undiscovered treasures. First, let's discuss the age-old practise of acupuncture. With the help of tiny needles and targeted body locations, my energy flow resumed immediately. Acupuncture not only helped with my nausea and exhaustion, but it also made me feel more balanced and at ease. It seemed like a journey inside of me, with breathing exercises and mindfulness practises serving as our tour guides and introspection and self-reflection as welcome guests.

There was also massage therapy. How powerful touch is! The strain fading away, delicious relief. My muscles were able to relax under the expert care of a therapist, and I experienced a profound sensation of harmony and tranquilly throughout my entire being. My haven, where I could release tension and let my body heal, was massage therapy.

However, the adventure didn't stop there, my friend. I delved into the world of mind-body techniques like yoga and meditation. Through these techniques, I was able to access my inner self. They nourished my soul by providing me with the means to control my tension and anxiety. I figured out the mysteries of who I was by sitting in silence and paying attention to my feelings and thoughts. I acquired a stronger comprehension and the fortitude to confront life's obstacles with lucidity.

Well, the mysteries of psychology! I discovered a psychologist with expertise in psychotherapy and coping mechanisms. I was able to delve deeply into the emotional and psychological toll the illness had taken on me because of the regular meetings. Together, we devised methods for stress management, self-compassion cultivation, and good mental development. During these sessions, I discovered the tremendous potential of a sound mind to aid in my recovery process.

My healing process became more than just physical and psychological as time went on. It turned into adopting a way of life that fed my entire self. I made self-care a priority and made time for joyful and soul-nourishing pursuits. My healing process included spending time with my loved ones, going on walks in the outdoors, writing in my diary, and using art and photography as a means of self-expression.

I never felt alone on this road, my buddy, let me tell you that. I discovered a group of people who shared my beliefs and who could relate to my struggles. We shared our experiences, gave each other advice, and provided encouragement to one another in support groups and online discussion boards. These relationships gave me comfort and a fresh lease on life.

Thus, here I am, thinking back on this amazing road to recovery. My heart is full with gratitude for the life-changing encounters that put me on the road to recovery. I not only successfully treated Hepatitis E by adopting a healthy diet, investigating holistic therapies, and emphasising self-care, but I also had a renewed sense of vitality and well-being. My friend, it was a voyage of self-discovery and resiliency that has permanently altered my perspective on fitness and health.

Let's now turn the page, my friend, and go more deeply into the particular methods and approaches that helped me on my path to recovery. I aim to provide insightful analysis and useful advice for properly managing hepatitis E. Together, we will investigate the effectiveness of coping mechanisms, self-care routines, counselling and psychology-related approaches, and a plethora of other topics. My goal is to enable you to take control of your own path to full management of Hepatitis E and recovery of your health with each page turn. Let us proceed!

The Power of Mind-Body Connection

It's amazing how our bodies function, you know. There's some really intricate stuff going on there. And here's the thing: it has also completely entangled our minds. Our physical health and general well-being can be severely harmed by our ideas, feelings, and even beliefs. Similar to how ancient healing systems understood the mind-body connection long before science did.

That's right, science is finally catching up and validating what those prehistoric guys already knew. Studies have demonstrated that our thoughts can disrupt our DNA, endocrine system, and immune system. Like, our minds are so powerful. Positive emotions and joyful thoughts release neuropeptides, which are substances that facilitate communication between the brain and body. And you know what? These neuropeptides support health, aid in healing, and maintain homeostasis inside the body. Really cool, huh?

Hold on, though; this is the other side. Emotions and beliefs that are negative can seriously damage us. Not to be laughed at. Our health suffers when we're always worried, tense, or depressed. Numerous chronic illnesses, including diabetes, cancer, and heart issues have all been connected to it. It's all due to the hormone cortisol, which is released under stressful conditions and drives us crazy. Additionally, a persistent excess of cortisol compromises our immune system, disrupts our digestive processes, and interferes with a host of other physiological processes.

But here's the thing, buddy. It's amazing how thinking positively may improve our health. It really can make a difference, like. Positive thinking has been shown to strengthen the immune system, reduce the risk of illness, and expedite the healing process. Crazy, you say? Still, a number of high-caliber studies support it, so you know it's real.

Furthermore, mindfulness plays a significant role in the mind-body connection game. We can learn to simply be in the present without passing judgement on our ideas or ourselves by practising mindfulness. We seem to become more aware of our true selves and our bodies. A large component of this is meditation. And it really does wonders, I tell you. It relaxes us, improves our quality of sleep, lessens the intensity of our discomfort, and generally makes us feel better. You have to try it, my friend.

And let's not overlook the importance of visualising. Here's where we visualise what we want to happen in our minds by using our imagination. For example, when we picture ourselves in perfect health and feeling wonderful, our body receives the message and begins to activate its innate healing abilities. It's crazy, yet science has also confirmed it. In fact, visualisation can strengthen our immune systems, lessen pain, and even improve our athletic performance. Did anyone think?

I have to tell you a few personal stories now. In my capacity as a physician and health coach, I have witnessed some astounding instances of this mind-body link in action. Really, I have seen patients who have entirely changed their lives via the use of visualisation, mindfulness, and positive thinking. It's not just me, either. My incredible group of health and wellness professionals is travelling with me. We go over everything, including nutrition planning, therapy, and self-care, as well as lifestyle adjustments. Our mission is to enable individuals to take charge of their health and utilise the mind-body connection. You have to personally experience it.

In summary, this mind-body phenomenon is astounding. Our beliefs, feelings, and attitudes have a profound effect on our health. It functions as a kind of manual for leading a fierce life and being an absolute badass. We have the secret weapons to unlock the mind-body link and become the healthiest versions of ourselves:

positive thinking, mindfulness, and visualisation. My buddy, it's a trip, but one that is well worth the effort.

Self-Care: Nurturing the Soul

The news that I had Hepatitis E struck me like a tonne of bricks. I felt all of a sudden that my standard medical training was not up to the task at hand. I was aware that I required an alternative strategy, one that would take into account all facets of my identity, including my emotional and spiritual aspects in addition to my physical ailments.

I've spent many years helping others on their own healing journeys as a doctor and health coach. It was now time for me to heed my own counsel. To help me get better from this awful sickness, I assembled a group of professionals from various wellness and health-related sectors, and we developed a self-care plan together.

Setting aside time for calming rituals was one of the first things I did every day. I am referring to the entire spa experience, which includes soothing massages, warm baths, and aromatherapy. It gave me bodily comfort, but it also served as a gentle reminder to calm down and look after my needs.

However, self-care went beyond taking care of my physical needs. I also discovered how crucial relaxation and rest are. I started paying attention to what my body required and allowed myself to decline anything that would tyre me out. Taking naps, cuddling up with a book, or just spending time alone myself were essential components of my daily schedule.

And believe me when I say that self-care encompasses far more than just physical well-being. It's about taking care of both your spirit and your emotions. That meant doing things that made me happy and relying on my loved ones for support. It made all the difference to be surrounded by folks who sympathised with my situation and uplifted me.

I experimented with a variety of self-help methods to help me heal as well. I used journaling, affirmations, and meditation to access my inner resilience and strength. Through these exercises, I was able to develop a positive outlook and let go of any negative feelings or ideas that were preventing me from moving forward.

My self-care ritual quickly turned into a sacred period of time when I could finally give myself the love and attention I so sorely needed. Every ritual and practise turned into an expression of self-compassion and self-love. It served as a reminder to myself that I was deserving of recovery and that my wellbeing was important.

And what's this? As I proceeded with my self-care journey, I saw some amazing shifts. My physical symptoms started to go away. I felt alive again and had more energy. I had a calm, grounded emotional state. I also experienced a strong sense of purpose and connection on a spiritual level.

Actually, studies have indicated that self-care routines can significantly improve our general wellbeing. They can strengthen our emotional and mental wellbeing, lessen stress, build resilience, and improve our physical health. We're not only taking care of ourselves when we prioritise self-care; we're also encouraging others to follow our lead.

We don't need to reserve self-care for rare occasions or as a luxury. It's a dedication to our wellbeing and an essential component of our everyday life. We are investing in our own recovery and strengthening our bonds with the people and things in our lives when we take care of our souls.

I thus wish to extend an invitation to you to start your own self-care path. Investigate the rituals that you find meaningful and incorporate them into your daily routine. Make rest and relaxation a priority, engage in calming rituals, rely on your loved ones, and discover self-help methods that you truly connect with. You can experience self-transformational love's power and grow stronger, more resilient, and more in tune with who you are by taking care of your soul.

The Importance of Self-Compassion

Allow me to share a little anecdote with you about something I've witnessed repeatedly in both my role as a health and wellness consultant and my medical practise. It's the detrimental impacts that self-criticism has on people's emotional and physical health. In particular, I've found that people who have Hepatitis E frequently turn against themselves. They blame themselves for not recovering entirely and beat themselves up for getting the infection. Furthermore, it's not helping them in any way, believe me.

We now need to dissect the idea of self-compassion into three components in order to comprehend it. First, practise self-compassion. That entails being kind and understanding to ourselves when times are difficult. We must learn to speak to ourselves with kindness and encouragement, just as we would to a close friend or loved one, rather than criticising and belittling ourselves for not living up to our standards.

Next is shared humanity. We must never forget that we are not experiencing our problems alone. Numerous individuals are experiencing the same problem as you. It's simpler to forgive ourselves and let go of self-judgment when we accept that our suffering and failures are merely a part of being human.

And last, thoughtful acceptance. It basically comes down to witnessing our feelings and ideas without resistance or judgement. It is important for us to learn how to be in pain or suffering without reacting or passing judgement. Practice is necessary, but it's worthwhile. Believe me.

Allow me to now share Sarah's tale with you. This young lady, who is fighting Hepatitis E, got off to a very bad start. She continually chastised herself for not being able to fully recover from the infection and blamed herself for catching it. And believe me when I say that her mental health suffered greatly as a result of her negative self-talk. She felt helpless and stressed out.

But when Sarah learned to be compassionate with herself, things began to shift. It was as clear as day to her that she had to treat herself with kindness and understanding. So she gradually changed her perspective. She began to give herself a break and stopped berating herself. She let go of all that self-judgment and praised even the smallest progress. It felt as though a burden had been removed from her.

And it continued after that. Sarah came to understand the value of self-care in her recovery process. She made time for the activities that made her happy, such as interacting with her loved ones, being creative, and spending time in nature. It was about putting herself and her health first, not just taking a break. And believe me when I say that there was a huge difference.

Sarah's experience is just one of many that demonstrate how treating Hepatitis E with self-compassion can change our approach. It all comes down to breaking down the barriers caused by self-criticism and developing a loving, supportive bond with ourselves. Because we make decisions that genuinely promote our wellbeing when we act from a position of love and understanding.

Thus, how can we begin putting self-compassion into practise in our own lives? Well, there are a few doable tactics that we can attempt. We can start by creating a daily self-compassion practise. We could attempt affirmations, journaling, or meditation. These exercises provide us a dedicated period of time to be with ourselves and cultivate our self-compassion.

Having a supportive community around us is another crucial tactic. People that support us and are aware of our struggles are what we need. It could be friends, family, support networks, or even virtual groups. When we share our path with like-minded folks, we receive validation and the necessary motivation to maintain our self-compassion.

Let's now discuss how to reframe self-defeating thoughts. Everybody has an inner critic that enjoys picking apart and criticising yourself. But we are able to respond. We might consciously choose to replace those pessimistic ideas with encouraging words. We can say things like, "I'm making improvement every day, and I'm damn proud of it," rather than, "I'm a failure because I haven't totally recovered."

Last but not least, self-care is essential. It's an essential component of self-love. We need to be doing things that feed our bodies, minds, and souls. It serves as a reminder that we deserve affection and attention. Self-care provides us the energy we need to develop that self-compassion, whether that means finding professional support, engaging in leisure activities, or simply taking some time to unwind.

Ultimately, the secret to recovering from hepatitis E is self-compassion. We may approach this chronic condition with compassion and grace when we practise mindful acceptance, accept ourselves as we are, and realise our common problems. My friend, you're not travelling alone in this adventure. Let's cultivate that self-compassion and have a happy, contented life.

Unleashing Inner Strength: Overcoming Obstacles

As a physician and health coach, I have witnessed some pretty awful things, man. Similar to the horrible disease Hepatitis E, which can truly debilitate a person. Whoa, what now? And I was struck by it. The experience like a gut-punch. As the saying goes, you have to look within yourself to find inner strength when life throws you curveballs. I carried out precisely that.

I resolved not to let this virus to define who I was. Not at all! I therefore began to focus on strengthening my resilience. As it happens, developing resilience is a necessary skill that cannot be acquired naturally. I so began to practise challenging things like journaling, deep breathing exercises, and meditation. The experience was akin to teaching my body and mind to maintain composure among the various challenges presented by Hepatitis E.

However, my friend, that's not all. Positive thought also proved to be powerful for me. My reality may be shaped by my ideas, I discovered. "I am strong and resilient," and "I am healing and bright," were some of the things I began telling myself. As corny as that may seem, it really did the trick. In those gloomy days, it gave me hope and completely changed my outlook.

Allow me to share with you my storey of appreciation, dude. Such material serves as spiritual fuel. Counting my blessings changed my perspective from dwelling on all the negative aspects of having Hepatitis E. Writing down three things for which I was thankful every day was my habit. A nice cup of coffee or a sunny day were examples of minor pleasures at times. Even with all the awful symptoms, though, those small things brought me happiness.

My primary concern shifted to taking care of myself. Because I was accustomed to putting other people before myself as a doctor, it wasn't easy. However, it dawned on me that neglecting my own needs would prevent me from being able to assist others. Consequently, I began engaging in joyful activities such as hiking, practising yoga, and engaging in my favourite pastimes. and relying on family and friends for support? That truly changed the game. I was able to continue because of their love, compassion, and support.

Nevertheless, my friend, I didn't finish there. In addition, I looked for supplementary and alternate methods. In addition to giving me more energy, acupuncture helped me manage the pain. What about those vitamins and natural cures? I felt like they boosted my immunity. Being actively involved in my recovery process felt good.

Tell you what, though, there were times when I wanted to give up. It demoralised and overwhelmed me. But Hepatitis E could not prevail over me. I regarded obstacles as chances for improvement even though I understood they were a necessary element of the game. I used every obstacle as an opportunity to show myself that I was resilient, strong, and capable of conquering any challenge.

Ah, man, you're going to get some real bad luck in life. How you manage it, though, is up to you. We are all incredibly strong, as my experience with Hepatitis E has shown me. Whatever the challenge, we have the ability to overcome it. That being said, I want you to know that you are capable of overcoming this infection. As you take care of yourself, find gratitude in the little things, start strengthening your resilience, and repeat positive affirmations to yourself. It's also a good idea to try out different approaches as you never know what you might find out. Okay, buddy, let's get started. Give Hepatitis E a run for its money and regain control of the disease.

Embracing the Power of Community

You know, after years of being a doctor and living life, I've witnessed something truly remarkable happen in front of my eyes: the remarkable influence that a person's community can have on their overall wellbeing. It resembles this strong force that has the ability to affect good changes in both the physical and emotional domains.

Permit me to share a storey with you that truly resonated with me. It's about Emma, a young lady. She was found to have hepatitis E, and let me tell you, getting well wasn't easy for her. She had suffered so much from the illness that her spirit had been crushed. But what's the deal? Emma was not alone in facing it. Making connections with people who had experienced like difficulties brought her comfort.

Emma joined this specialised support group for hepatitis E patients. She discovered something genuinely unique there, in that secure environment: others who shared her anxieties, disappointments, and even triumphant moments. It served as a sort of lifeline for her recovery. Emma felt suddenly that she was not alone. She had found a group of people who understood her hardships and were exactly like her.

Emma found both practical guidance and emotional solace in that support group, though. Group members discussed new treatments, coping mechanisms, and even lifestyle adjustments that had been successful for them. Emma felt as though she had discovered a goldmine of information that would enable her to actively participate in her own care and have a deeper understanding of her illness.

Not to be overlooked are the amazing medical professionals Emma met along the way. They were friends and allies in addition to being skilled medical professionals. Emma felt not alone because of their consistent support, encouragement, and ability to listen. Together, they worked nonstop to support her recovery.

The problem is that it goes beyond support networks and medical experts. It's about the people who are in our life all the time: our family, friends, and loved ones. Their steadfast assistance might significantly impact our recuperation process. Emma was fortunate to have a family who assisted her with daily chores when she was physically ill in addition to providing emotional support. Her general well-being was much enhanced by their presence, which gave her a sense of security and served as a reminder that she was loved.

Studies have confirmed what I have personally seen: community support does, in fact, improve health outcomes. Research has indicated that those with strong social networks or access to support groups heal more quickly and have less symptoms. According to one study, those with long-term illnesses who experienced high levels of social support also experienced reduced mortality rates.

How can you, then, harness the strength of your community to further your own healing process? You must first actively seek out and call out for support. Participate in support groups, consult medical professionals for advice, and, with the help of technology, you may even establish online connections with people experiencing similar circumstances. There are apps for wellness and mental health that provide virtual support; you have options, my buddy.

Additionally, remember how important it is to have a network of family and friends who are able to provide that companionship and emotional support. Not only does opening up to trustworthy friends and family help reduce feelings of loneliness, but it also provides a channel for sincere understanding and connection. They might be your partners in putting new lifestyle adjustments or self-care routines into action, or they can just be that listening ear.

The worst part is that community support is a two-way street. You have the ability to change someone else's life, just as others can aid in your own recovery process. Giving back creates a genuine sense of community spirit and a profound sense of fulfilment. Examples of this include lending a helping hand to someone in need and sharing your experiences to inspire others.

So keep this in mind, my friend: your recovery process can be greatly aided by embracing the power of community. You can establish relationships with people who can offer consolation, information, and encouragement through support groups, medical professionals, and the love and understanding of your loved ones. The empathy and shared experiences of others become a beacon in the darkness, and healing becomes a group endeavour. Accept the strength of your community and allow it to help you achieve both full hepatitis E management and a healthy, happy life.

Nurturing Relationships

The Fragile Bonds of Friendship

Man, friendships are like our lives' GPS systems. They provide us companionship, support, and a feeling of community. However, let me assure you that these friendships can be severely tested when it comes to managing Hepatitis E. It can be especially difficult to tell your friends the truth about your disease since you're afraid of being judged and stigmatised. You can seriously doubt yourself since you never know how they're going to respond.

You know, I'll never forget that first encounter. That was the day I had to tell one of my best friends the truth. Man, it seemed like you were walking a tightrope. Even though we had known each other for ages, I couldn't help but wonder how they would respond. Would they retreat gradually, as if to say, "Oh no, this is too much for me"? Would they begin to handle me like I was made of china? I was mentally preparing myself for that conversation like it was a flipping carnival.

Now, though, what? My friend turned out to be a rock star, surprise, surprise. They addressed me directly and stated, "Hey, our bond is far more resilient than any illness. No matter what, I've got your back." I was able to breathe once more in an instant. My concerns had been unfounded, and if anything, our relationship became closer. I learned a lot from that experience, man. It made me realise how important it is to be forthright and honest with our friends about our health issues. It enables them to empathise with us and support us throughout our most trying times.

However, let's face it—not every friendship has a happily ever after. Not everyone will understand the nature of Hepatitis E and how it affects our day-to-day existence. They might merely back off out of fear, or they might say stupid things without realising it. My buddy, it's crucial to handle certain circumstances with tolerance and compassion. Give them time to learn about it all and make sense of it all.

Man, I've been there. Some of my pals didn't fully understand the implications of having Hepatitis E. Sometimes they would ask me why I looked like I got hit by a bus, or they would invite me to parties without considering the risks. I told them how the condition affects my energy levels and general well-being, although it required some time and effort. You know, sometimes you just have to put it out for them. It's a two-way street as well. Man, we have to be honest about our needs and limitations. Tell them how they can help us effectively. Telling them about the illness or letting them know when we need a break to refuel could be necessary.

However, we also need to be understanding and patient with our friends. Not everyone will comprehend everything at once. They have their own challenges, worries, and misconceptions. Let them have some time to come to terms with the new normal of our friendship. It's like to breaking in new shoes; it will eventually fit perfectly, but it takes some getting used to.

Alright, so here's the deal about friendships and all. We may go into self-imposed hibernation mode as a result of hepatitis E. The stigma attached to this sickness by society makes us want to curl up in a hole and never come out. We fear rejection, judgement, and other negative outcomes. Therefore, we cut ourselves off from the very friendships that could encourage us and provide us with a positive boost.

Man, I've seen it happen. Its seclusion resembles a black hole. It causes a great deal of hopelessness, misery, and loneliness. That being said, it's important for us to remember that humans are more than merely machines capable of disease. All those rewarding friendships are ours, no more, no less. We need to surround ourselves with a strong support network of friends who appreciate and understand us for who we are. Seek out those who are either willing to learn about Hepatitis E or who genuinely understand what it is. You know, those people could end up being our secret society, our wingmen. In a secure environment, we can talk about our worries, ideas, and experiences. We'll travel this route together, encouraging and supporting one another all the way.

In summary, it's difficult to make and maintain friends while you have Hepatitis E. Fear of being judged and stigmatised can seriously damage our mental health. But guy, we have to be honest with our pals. We need to be transparent with them about our health issues. While some friendships may be put to the test, others may simply grown stronger as a result of everything. We may cultivate and preserve such significant friendships by being honest, establishing boundaries, and surrounding ourselves with a network of support. Recall that this condition does not define who we are. We deserve amazing friendships that support and uplift us as we navigate this wild life.

Love in the Time of Hepatitis E

Greetings from the "Love in the Time of Hepatitis E" section. I'm going to delve into the fascinating realm of love partnerships in which one spouse has this illness. Get ready for real insights and poignant tales that will change your perspective on love.

For a moment, let's discuss the power of love. Is that not all-conquering? However, things become a little trickier when Hepatitis E comes into play. All of a sudden, love requires a lot of empathy, a generous helping of comprehension, and an open exchange of communications to function. Now, these characteristics become even more important for couples navigating the ups and downs of Hepatitis E infection.

The fear of transmission is one of the main obstacles that couples encounter in these circumstances. Contaminated water, food, and even sexual intercourse can transmit hepatitis E. You can only image the level of anxiety this may put the partner without the disease through. It appears as though a gloomy cloud is threatening to spoil their connection.

Allow me to recount John and Sarah's tale (names changed to protect their privacy). They were among the couples who contacted me in search of advice. Sarah was having a hard time accepting the news that John had been diagnosed with hepatitis E. Despite their intense love and bond, Hepatitis E seemed to want to be the antagonist in their romance.

We thus had some heart-to-heart talks and encouraged them to share their emotions, worries, and hopes. You see, effective communication is essential to any successful partnership. However, it takes on even greater significance when it comes to couples who are coping with hepatitis E. We needed to figure out how to promote closeness and connection while reducing the chance of transmission.

I cannot emphasise enough how important it was for John and Sarah to prioritise hepatitis E education and awareness. This was my first piece of advice to them. Their ability to control their concerns and make wise judgments increased with their knowledge of symptoms, prevention, and modes of transmission. Equipped with this understanding, they could establish a secure and encouraging environment for their love to grow.

And then there was the crucial subject of safe sex, my friends. Well, I'm not claiming that hepatitis E is extremely frequent to spread sexually, but it's always best to be safe than sorry. We therefore discussed integrating safer sexual practices—such as regular condom use—into their private moments. It not only lessened the chance of transmission but also offered comfort and security to both partners.

However, we must not overlook the sentimental side of love. It can be difficult to maintain one's mental and emotional health while dealing with a chronic illness like hepatitis E, which can have an impact on a relationship. I therefore advised them to put emotional support and self-care first in their relationship.

For John, this meant going to therapy in order to deal with any fear or anguish that his diagnosis might be causing him. He acquired coping mechanisms in treatment to control his emotions and maintain an optimistic view on life. Regarding Sarah, I suggested that she seek assistance from a therapist or attend a support group intended especially for spouses of people with long-term diseases. She would have a secure place to voice her worries and fears and receive advice on how to handle their particular circumstance.

There should always be a reciprocal flow of support and compassion between spouses. John and Sarah came to appreciate the value of supporting one another emotionally, understanding one another, and showing one another unconditional love. They realised that love could overcome all obstacles and that their relationship was not defined by Hepatitis E.

Together, they learned the value of resiliency and flexibility on their path. They accepted dietary and physical activity regimens as well as other lifestyle modifications that would improve their overall health and wellbeing. Together, they forged a stronger link and prioritised their general well-being by implementing these modifications.

When I think back on relationships like John and Sarah, I can't help but be amazed at the possibility of love even in the face of hardship. Undoubtedly, Hepatitis E presents certain difficulties. However, it should never take precedence over the potential for a happy and caring partnership. Couples can successfully manage the complications of Hepatitis E by encouraging open communication, engaging in safe sexual behaviour, getting emotional support, and placing a high priority on self-care.

We have explored the complex realm of romantic relationships when one person has Hepatitis E in this section. We have discussed the particular difficulties that these couples have encountered and offered helpful suggestions on how to establish and maintain a strong relationship through moving tales and open introspection. By the time this is through, I hope you will have gained a better understanding of the mental and physical dimensions of love in the context of Hepatitis E, as well as some practical tips for creating closeness and connection. My friends, even in the era of Hepatitis E, love remains unrivalled. And couples can succeed on their journey together if they have the correct resources and assistance.

The Family Tapestry

I've seen everything. As a physician and wellness coach, I have seen firsthand the emotional rollercoaster that can rip a family apart when Hepatitis E strikes. I can assure you that it's not a pleasant sight. Tension, fear, and confusion—it feels like a pressure cooker on the verge of blowing up.

One patient, Sarah, for example, came to me looking for comfort during the height of her Hepatitis E episode. Her family was like a rock for her at first. However, as time passed, fissures were visible. Sarah's parents overprotected their lovely daughter in a desperate bid to keep her safe. Their incessant pestering about medication, food, and avoiding anything that could cause a flare-up had her feeling like a fly on rice. Their love was what kept them going, but in the end, it choked Sarah to death and stifled the environment at home.

But don't worry, I'm here to offer you the dirt on how to deal with this outbreak of Hepatitis E. So fasten your seatbelts and get ready for some insightful tales and advice. Even in the deepest moments, we will make amends, transform the conflict into strength, and allow the love to prevail.

First things first, buddy: talk to each other. It's essential to maintaining family harmony in these unsettling times. Take a seat, have a private conversation, and reveal everything. Talk about your hopes, worries, and fears. Ensure that everyone is aware of the situation and is on the same page. I promise that expressing yourself fully and being open will greatly improve the tense family dynamic.

What did I take away from Sarah's experience, you ask? Ah, education. Understanding is power. The dawn dawned on Sarah's parents as they learned all about Hepatitis E, including how it spreads and how to nurture their daughter without becoming overbearing. It dawned on them at last that Sarah could take care of her own health, with them acting as her support system. And then love took over the reins, and their entire family started to feel like they were on Christmas morning.

Hold on, family. The emotional toll that hepatitis E has on all parties involved is something we cannot overlook. It like an ominous cloud hanging over your head, threatening to spoil your plans. That's where my ability to provide psychological support becomes useful. I'm not just a medical wizard—I'm also your support system on an emotional level.

My arsenal of skills includes mindfulness meditation. Shut your eyes, inhale deeply, and embrace the present moment. Finding inner peace and making sense of the turbulent emotions around your head are made easier with mindfulness. It's also like a peaceful symphony that replaces fear with thankfulness and fortitude when done as a family.

Oh, and one thing I really want to emphasise is self-care. Friend, watch out for yourself. This is a cooperative effort rather than a solo endeavour. Cherish the little things in life, take pauses when necessary, and rely on supportive friends and family. Because, in a way, your life depends on it, avoid burnout as much as possible.

The truth is that hepatitis E can either destroy families or strengthen them beyond recognition. It all comes down to how you approach those obstacles. Discuss it, share knowledge, and look after one another. You will create a link with each other that will endure earthquakes, hurricanes, and all other calamities in life.

Hepatitis E, you see, is more than just a disease. It's an opportunity for resilience, empathy, and growth. It teaches us to cherish the present, be gentler to ourselves and others, and rely on the love that is all around us. As you delve deeper into the book, stop to consider the dynamics in your own family. Allow the anecdotes and guidance to flow into your spirit and meld with your life. Keep in mind that this is a family issue rather than just your battle.

Now let's go kick Hepatitis E's butt, one hug at a time.

Finding Support in Unlikely Places

I discovered early on in my Hepatitis E journey that support can come from the most surprising places. Let me tell you, making connections with people who have gone through similar things may really transform your life. In this section, I want to go further into the significance of these relationships and examine the various ways that we soldiers with Hepatitis E can look for and welcome supportive networks. I promise you that these relationships allow us to be resilient, strong, and find comfort when faced with hardship.

My friend, let's begin with the virtual community. These days, the internet is like a lifeline to us. It resembles a desert oasis. Our online community of compassion and understanding has taken the form of forums and support groups. Upon initially exploring these virtual communities, I was astounded by the abundance of wisdom and empathy that awaited me on the other side of the screen.

Envision this: people from diverse backgrounds, confronting similar challenges, uniting and offering resolute assistance. It resembles magic. These virtual networks turn into our forum for exchanging narratives, posing queries, and obtaining consolation on an emotional level. And let me tell you something, my friend: it's a comforting balm for the spirit to know that you're not travelling alone.

Numerous motivational stories that demonstrate the strength of these virtual relationships have come across my path. Sarah, a young lady, was informed that she had Hepatitis E while she was pregnant. Can you imagine how alone and overwhelmed she felt? worrying all the time about the health of her unborn child. Now, though, what? Sarah was able to locate other pregnant women who had experienced similar difficulties by means of an internet support group. They provided not just emotional support but also useful guidance on controlling the problem during pregnancy, akin to guardian angels. Sarah's newly formed network served as her pillar of support, enabling her to confront her diagnosis with fortitude and resolve.

Let's now discuss the therapeutic value of in-person support groups. My friend, I'm talking about in-person conversations. People who are aware of your situation get together in those spaces, and there's an indisputable energy there. Hepatitis E support groups offer a secure environment in which we may connect and exchange our stories, anxieties, and successes. The stories that are freely shared in those communities are gold, I promise you. They infuse the atmosphere with inspiration and hope. It is similar to inhaling bravery.

Imagine a collection of people, each at a different point in their Hepatitis E experience, each providing unique viewpoints and thoughts. We take comfort in the knowledge that we're not alone when we band together. We can rely on the assistance and guidance of those who have overcome comparable obstacles. When we feel like we're drowning, it's like a lifeline that's always there to help us surface, my friend.

Let's now explore the realm of complementary and alternative therapies communities. Here, we examine novel methods of healing. In addition to relieving physical problems, acupuncture, yoga, meditation, and herbal therapies offer a strong sense of emotional and psychological support. I can attest to the transformational impact of these therapies, my friend. Trust me.

Consider David as an example. He was dissatisfied with traditional therapies and had been struggling with Hepatitis E for years. However, he later discovered a society devoted to acupuncture. And boy, did that affect his life. He learned about acupuncture's amazing healing powers as he related his experiences to his newfound group. It provided him with relief unlike anything he had ever felt before and encouraged his body's innate healing capabilities.

And what's this? This group also served as a source of emotional support. The difference was immense when he found folks who genuinely understood his challenges.

But, my friend, here's the thing. Support can occasionally appear in the most unexpected places. Imagine meeting someone by coincidence who also happens to have your condition, or having a fortuitous chat with a buddy you never expected to support you. These times have a certain kind of enchantment, my friend. They serve as a reminder that even in the most improbable places, we can find understanding and connection.

Allow me to introduce you to Emily, a patient who had been handling her Hepatitis E treatment on her own. Because she was afraid of their disbelief and lack of understanding, she never felt comfortable telling her loved ones about her illness. However, she chose to tell her nurse about her problem during a standard check-up. And you know what? The nurse had, it turned out, gone through something similar herself. Is it really true? The two women supported and mentored one another through their same hardships as their unexpected friendship flourished.

So, my friend, this is what I've discovered on my own journey: in order to find support, we need to keep an open mind and be willing to accept the unexpected. You can never be sure where it will originate. Even if it could just be a brief exchange of words or a simple discussion, those relationships, my friend, have the power to genuinely transform. It all comes down to exposing ourselves and moving past our comfort zones. That's the location of the magic.

To sum up, my fellow warriors, in order to maintain our resilience and general well-being while coping with Hepatitis E, we must look for assistance in unexpected places. A large network of empathy and understanding is available online, support groups offer in-person spaces for us to share our stories, and alternative and complementary therapy communities offer comprehensive approaches to recovery. Above all, though, we have to learn to welcome the unexpected. Genuine relationships are capable of overcoming all obstacles, and we can receive help in unexpected ways.

So, my friend, let's look for these encouraging networks. Come together with others that genuinely get our path and let's uncover the power and resilience that lay within each of us. Because, as always, we are never alone ourselves. One of the most potent forces we have is each other. With the help of one another and the understanding that sometimes appears in the most unexpected places, we can overcome the difficulties associated with controlling hepatitis E.

The Healing Power of Compassion

I can assure you that managing Hepatitis E is not a simple task. You feel as though you've been knocked down and dragged through the mud as a result of it, both physically and emotionally. You may start to doubt everything because it's a solitary struggle. The truth is, though, people: even in the worst of times, kindness can shine brightly.

I've personally witnessed it with my patients. Consider the case of Sarah. After receiving the Hepatitis E diagnosis, she entered my clinic a bundle of nerves and fear. Her deep-seated grief and longing for someone to simply understand it were seen in her eyes.

We had a heart-to-heart once we sat down. It's acceptable to feel angry, irritated, and depressed, I had to explain to her. Such feelings are expected in the area. However, treating yourself with kindness and a little sympathy is just as vital. We discussed journaling, mindfulness meditation, positive affirmations, and self-care practises as well as other methods that could help her feel better.

It didn't end there, though. I informed her about John, a different patient of mine, who took solace in his family's kindness. He shared his journey with his loved ones and chose to accept his fear rather than run from it. And my goodness, did their love and encouragement pay off. It did more than only deepen their relationship; it also somewhat eased John's struggle.

It is a two-way street, my friends, compassion. The dance is reciprocal. We provide a safe space for people to talk about their challenges when we approach them with a modicum of empathy and compassion. What do you know? On their path to recovery, that affirmation and connection can perform wonders.

Maria is another patient of mine who I would like to present to you. When the poor thing was diagnosed with hepatitis E, she felt alone and ashamed. She kept it a secret out of fear that her friends would condemn and reject her. But then she happened into a warrior support group where other warriors were engaged in the same conflict. What did she discover there, do you know? a feeling of acceptance. a neighbourhood that accepted her as she was. It offered her the confidence to confide in her friends and seek their help. And believe me when I say that the kindness she encountered helped her to overcome her guilt and realised she wasn't fighting this battle alone.

Folks, this is what I learned. Empathy has a revolutionary effect. Hepatitis E patients must take care of themselves and ask for support from their loved ones. Accelerating the healing process requires building an understanding community.

You want additional evidence, too? Shall we begin our investigation now? Compassion practise has been demonstrated in studies to enhance both mental and physical well-being. According to one study, those who practise self-compassion have decreased rates of anxiety and despair. According to a different Stanford University study, compassion activates the same brain regions as are activated by a pat on the back: the reward centres. Now, I'm not sure what more scientific proof there is for the therapeutic value of compassion if that.

In summary, guys, showing compassion to people who have Hepatitis E can be rather beneficial. The key is to practise self-compassion and to share that compassion with others. We can establish a supportive, restorative, and community atmosphere by working together. The anecdotes I have provided here help to remind people that kindness has the power to transform lives—both of persons who are afflicted with Hepatitis E and of those who support them. In order to manage Hepatitis E, embrace compassion and observe how it changes your path and the wonderful connections you make along the route.

From Surviving to Thriving

A Glimpse of Darkness

It all began with a standard hospital check-up. I merely assumed that my hectic work schedule was the reason behind my constant fatigue and sporadic stomachaches. Whoa, I was incorrect. As it happened, those symptoms were only the beginning. The doctor's face turned pale and his voice took on a serious tone as soon as he saw my test results. He said, "You have Hepatitis E," and it felt like he had just given me the death penalty.

My head began to spin, and I had trouble breathing. Thoughts of fear and perplexity seized over as my surroundings became indistinct. How in the world am I the victim of this? I advocate for balanced lifestyles, self-care, and healthy living. How did I come to have a possibly fatal illness?

And thus the adventure on the rollercoaster started. I had to confront my mental and physical suffering head-on. My diagnosis of hepatitis E came as a huge blow. Every movement felt like a battle because my body felt like it had been crushed by a huge vehicle. My constant companions became nausea, exhaustion, and this awful fever that would not go away. The nights, though, were the worst. My body was in excruciating pain in the darkness, and thoughts of an uncertain future tormented my head.

However, the bodily suffering was only half the fight. My mental health was also being negatively impacted by hepatitis E. Anxiety and depression started to seem like unwanted intruders who took away my joy and sapped my energy. The bright, cheerful me of old was engulfed by shadows. I had the impression that I was drowning in a sea of hopelessness and was completely alone.

I eventually realised the value of self-care and adopting the proper mindset during those difficult times. Yes, I had preached about it for years, but it was time for me to put my words into action. For advice and assistance, I therefore went to my team of professionals from several health and wellness domains. They gave me a tonne of tools and strategies to help me get through the most difficult parts of my journey.

Making lifestyle adjustments a regular part of my routine was one of the game-changers. I came to understand how crucial it was to unwind and rest so that my body could recover and replenish itself. My haven of calm in the middle of the mayhem was meditation. I was able to find peace and quiet the unpleasant thoughts that were racing through my head by practising mindfulness.

Not to mention the importance of food. My team of specialists created a customised diet plan with the goal of providing my body with the nutrition it needs to combat Hepatitis E. As my accomplices in crime, fresh fruits and vegetables provided me with vital vitamins and antioxidants. Sustenance was more than simply food; it was now my medicine and a vital instrument in my recovery process.

The emotional obstacles necessitated professional assistance and treatment. I went to counselling in order to address the ingrained trauma and dread that had taken over my thoughts. By sharing my deepest feelings and ideas, I was able to release the pressure that had been holding me down. I began to regain strength and optimism as a result of these sessions.

I explored complementary therapies and alternative forms of self-care in addition to conventional therapy. I started receiving acupuncture and acupressure, which helped me feel better overall and get relief from physical pain. My go-to exercises became tai chi and yoga, which helped me let go of my physical strain. These techniques created new avenues for healing and restoration when paired with the healing potential of touch and energy healing.

The discovery of self-help methods and coping mechanisms, however, was one of the largest, most significant shifts in my journey. In an attempt to find inspiration and drive to keep moving forward,

I delved into self-help literature and went to personal development seminars. My perspective gradually changed from one of helplessness to one of empowerment. I came to understand that the darkness I had experienced may have strengthened and resilient me.

Now, when I reflect on those difficult times during my journey with hepatitis E, I can't help but be thankful. I gained a fresh perspective on life and a more profound comprehension of what it meant to be healthy during that period of extreme sadness. Yes, I did see a glimpse of darkness at the beginning of my journey, but finally I found the light.

Embracing Resilience

Guy, resilience. This attribute holds immense significance in situations where life presents unexpected challenges. It's the capacity to pick oneself up, adjust, and carry on when times are difficult. Furthermore, let me tell you that perseverance is like our collective hidden weapon when it comes to coping with Hepatitis E.

So, I've been lucky enough to meet some absolutely remarkable folks who have shown incredible tenacity in their battle with Hepatitis E. Consider Sarah as an example. When that diagnosis was made for her, she was just 25 years old. Could you envision? But Sarah chose to take charge of her life and embrace resilience, treating it like her own personal superhero sidekick, rather than allowing fear and uncertainty to control her.

Sarah began by being knowledgeable about her disease. From the symptoms to the available treatments, she was interested in learning everything there was to know about Hepatitis E. It's true that knowledge is power. She didn't stop there, either. Sarah made connections with people who were experiencing similar problems by contacting support groups. Her guiding light during the worst moments was the tenacity, hope, and success revealed in those stories. That type of help, guy, it really does make a difference.

However, what about Sarah truly caught my attention? She was very hopeful. She did not consider herself to be a HEV victim. She considered herself to be a fearless survivor, equipped to face any challenge that might arise. When things got difficult, she was able to find strength because of her optimistic outlook. And they got tough, I assure you.

Sarah also excelled at taking care of herself. She understood how critical it was to look after her mental, emotional, and physical health. She began eating well, exercising on a regular basis, and getting adequate sleep. And she made time for the activities that gave her happiness and calm, such as art therapy, meditation, and quality time with her family. Finding that balance and taking care of oneself from the inside out was crucial.

Here's the real deal, people. Sarah became aware of the value of self-compassion. Even when things didn't go according to plan, she was kind with herself. She accepted that obstacles were a necessary part of the process and allowed herself to grieve and recover. Man, that self-compassion was like a hidden weapon in her arsenal. She was able to handle the highs and lows of her trip with acceptance and grace because to it.

Sarah's tale is currently only one of many. There are a plethora of amazing people in the world who have overcome hardship and persevered despite the odds. They all have distinct histories, but they also have some characteristics and methods in common that we may all take note of.

like flexibility. You know how to roll with the punches when you're a resilient person? They are aware that there will be obstacles on the route of their recovery and that it is not a straight line. However, they view those detours as chances for learning and development rather than as reasons to feel bad about themselves.

Also, kids are aware of the importance of asking for help. establishing a network of people who will support and look out for them? It would be like to having your own cheer squad ready at all times. These relationships can be quite beneficial, whether they be for counselling, support groups, or just someone to vent to.

It doesn't end there, though. Reflecting on their experiences is something that resilient people do. They recognise their assets and use them as the cornerstones of their resiliency. Furthermore, they have no problem owning up to their shortcomings and working to improve them. It's all about that introspection and self-examination, dude.

So, let me explain. It takes a mental adjustment to embrace resilience in the face of hepatitis E. It entails making the decision to find hope at the darkest hours, to draw strength from vulnerability, and to acknowledge that setbacks may serve as stepping stones toward bigger things. It's about being open to the chances that present themselves, accepting the trip, and taking in the teachings.

I won't sugarcoat it, I promise. Hepatitis E is not an easy disease to treat. Nonetheless, we can discover the resilience within ourselves to not just survive but flourish if we can take a lesson from Sarah's and other people's experiences. Therefore, as we travel our own path toward resilience, let their stories serve as both an inspiration and a guide.

Together, my friends, we can overcome the difficulties caused by hepatitis E and discover the inner fortitude necessary to continue on. Strong will, dude. It is our covert armament. And with it, we're ready to face any challenge life presents.

The Gift of Gratitude

Shifting Perspective

It seemed as though the earth had split open and engulfed me completely when I was initially informed that I had Hepatitis E. I felt overwhelmed, apprehensive, and fearful. But all changed when I made the decision to fully immerse myself in the field of holistic healthcare and wellness. I learned from it that sometimes all you need is a change of viewpoint. I began looking for those bright spots rather than focusing on the drawbacks and difficulties of my illness. And believe me when when I say that's when I discovered the most priceless gift of all: appreciation.

Finding Gratitude in the Smallest Moments

Amidst the chaos that Hepatitis E brought into my life, I came upon something remarkable. Some tiny moments of plenty and beauty had found a way in, even in the midst of everything that looked dismal and dark. It may be anything as basic as the sight of a loved one smiling or the soothing warmth of a cup of tea in the morning. These little times, my friend, turned into my lifesaver. They served as a reminder that despite the difficulties I faced, blessings remained all around me just waiting to be acknowledged. You see, being grateful wasn't about acting like everything was fine. It was about shining a bright light on the gloom by accepting the good, no matter how tiny.

Embracing Joy and Healing

Now, let me tell you, everything changed once I accepted thankfulness totally as my go-to tactic for happiness and recovery. I started to understand that I could develop this amazing sense of hope and resilience within of me by concentrating on the positive things of my life. I was no longer just a patient with a Hepatitis E diagnosis. I was so much more than that, I swear. I had the ability to design a happy, meaningful life for myself. My friend, gratitude turned into a road to recovery that I was unable to keep to myself. I had a strong want to spread it to other people in order to illuminate their path to transformation.

Heartfelt Anecdotes and Reflective Musings

I welcome you to enter my world, which is replete with poignant tales and thoughtful reflections on my own experience with hepatitis E and thankfulness, throughout this chapter. I'll walk you through the times when I felt peace and contentment as a result of thankfulness pulling me up out of the deepest abysses of sorrow. These tales demonstrate, my friend, that despite how bad things may get, there is always something to be thankful for. Always.

Inviting Readers to Embrace Gratitude

We are currently on the latter part of our adventure together. And I must admit that I'm ecstatic to have you here. Now is the moment for me to reach out and provide an invitation to accept appreciation as your personal light during your journey with Hepatitis E. I'll provide you with some useful hints and activities to support the development of your personal thankfulness routine. I assure you that it's a worthwhile adventure. Hey, don't just believe what I say. I'll present you with the empirical evidence supporting the remarkable advantages of gratitude. My friend, this isn't simply some corny idea. It's a transformationally potent instrument that you may access.

Step-by-Step Guide:

1. Shifting Perspective

Let's explore in detail the effectiveness of changing our viewpoint as we navigate the path of hepatitis E. I'll talk about my personal experiences and how I overcame anxiety and uncertainty to feel grateful and hopeful. And I'll be by your side, supporting you to look past the obstacles and discover thankfulness in your own life.

2. Finding Gratitude in the Smallest Moments

Seize the moment, as we are about to uncover the enchantment of discovering thankfulness in the smallest of circumstances. I will share with you some of my personal tales, times when, in the midst of the tumultuous storm, I managed to find that flicker of appreciation. Hey, I'm not going to abandon you. I'll also provide you with some useful advice on how to develop your own thankfulness practise.

3. Embracing Joy and Healing

Prepare to discover the amazing relationship that exists between thankfulness and our general state of wellbeing. We will explore how cultivating that everlasting hope within us and how being grateful may help us overcome the most difficult circumstances. Our path together, my friend, is all about using the power of thankfulness to embrace joy and heal.

4. Heartfelt Anecdotes and Reflective Musings

Yes, it's time for a storey. I'll weave together heartfelt personal stories to show you how thankfulness changed my experience of living with hepatitis E. I'll think back to the times when thankfulness reached out to me, lifted me above the depths of hopelessness, and left me full of serenity. You'll realise how transformative appreciation can be by reading these stories.

5. Inviting Readers to Embrace Gratitude

Now, at the conclusion of our journey, here we are. But fear not—not it's truly the end. I'm here to provide an invitation to you to start a thankfulness journey. I'll provide you doable tasks and resources to help you get started on a thankfulness practise. Hey, I'll even pull out the big guns: factual evidence supporting every statement. So grab my hand, friend, and together we will enter this world of thankfulness that can improve your experience with Hepatitis E. Even in the most trying situations, there is hope, joy, and healing waiting for you—trust me. Allow this chapter to serve as your road map for maximising the amazing potential of thankfulness.

Unleashing the Growth Mindset

Let me tell you, having Hepatitis E is an incredible journey. Even just the physical symptoms might make you feel like a shell of the person you used to be. Not to mention the emotional toll and the never-ending uncertainty of what lies next. It's enough to give someone the impression that they're bearing the weight of the entire world.

But hear me out, buddy—I've come to see the benefits of having a development mentality. Let me tell you a brief tale from my own experience that made this incredibly clear to me. I had great intentions of becoming a top-notch physician a few years ago. I used to dream of working in a nice hospital, uniforms and all. But then—whoa! For me, fate had other ideas. It felt like my dreams were dissipating in front of me when I was unable to obtain a residency post in any prominent hospital.

I had to decide now what to do. I had two options: I could allow myself to be overcome by hopelessness and give up on my goals, or I could decide to use this setback as a chance to improve. And what's this? I went with the latter, and wow, did it change everything.

I threw myself into reading books on personal development, went to every conference I could find, and looked to mentors who had experience overcoming obstacles to achieve success. And believe me when I say that, although it wasn't simple, the difference was enormous. I came to understand that failure was merely a detour on the path to success—it did not define who I was. I began to have confidence in my own abilities and my capacity to get past any challenges I faced.

And believe me when I say that this mental adjustment has nothing to do with my work, my friend. It crept into every crevice of my existence. I began to understand that obstacles and hardships, be they related to Hepatitis E or otherwise, are opportunities for development rather than impediments. They support our growth in strength, flexibility, and resourcefulness.

Thus, using this way of thinking to the field of managing hepatitis E is revolutionary, don't you think? Look, I understand that having this illness can make you feel helpless and defeated. However, we may develop a sense of hope and take control of our own health and well-being by embracing a development mentality.

The idea that aptitude and intelligence can be acquired with perseverance and hard effort is fundamental to this way of thinking. It entails being aware that we can still actively work to enhance our health even if we have Hepatitis E. Things like maintaining a healthy diet, exercising frequently, controlling stress, and keeping up with new therapy developments.

I won't lie: having Hepatitis E necessitates extreme resilience and a growth-oriented mindset. It entails acknowledging the illness as real, addressing all of the associated feelings, and asking for help when we need it. However, it also entails dispelling those unfavourable notions and accepting the notion that we can thrive in spite of this diagnosis.

Here's a useful hint for you: Spend some time thinking about your advantages and the knowledge you've gained from having Hepatitis E. To serve as a constant reminder of your strength and capabilities, write them down and refer back to them often. And, hey, remember to build a toolkit of coping mechanisms. Make a point of including joyful, calming, and purposeful practises and activities into your everyday routine. Investing in your general well-being, whether it be through meditation, taking up a creative pastime, or going for a walk in the outdoors, positions you to develop and persevere.

Lastly, remember to surround yourself with a network of people who are supportive. Make connections with others who are aware of your experience, whether they are medical professionals who sincerely care about your well-being or other Hepatitis E warriors. I promise you, it makes all the difference to have allies.

In summary, my friend, the key to effectively controlling Hepatitis E is to have a growth attitude. It all comes down to having faith in our capacity to develop, learn, and adjust to whatever challenges life us. It gives us the ability to take charge of our health, develop resilience, and seize any chance for personal development that presents itself. Hepatitis E is not the death sentence when we adopt a growth attitude; rather, it is merely one more chapter in our narrative.

Rewriting the Narrative

I mean, I'm a health coach and a doctor, right? And let me tell you, I don't treat Hepatitis E the same way as most people. There's a lot more to it than just treating the physical symptoms, of course. Equally significant is the psychological and emotional aspect of the illness. The truth is that we can foster a culture of healing and development by altering the way we discuss hepatitis E. You know, it's like rewriting the entire script.

But first, we need to step back and assess our current situation. We may experience feelings of overwhelm, fear, and sometimes even humiliation when we have hepatitis E. Without a doubt, it's not easy. But the first step to writing our own narrative is acknowledging these feelings.

I therefore have a few aces in my sleeve to assist us in rewriting this storey. Among them is thankfulness. It really is a game-changer, I assure you. Our entire perspective changes when we begin to dwell on the things for which we are thankful. All of a sudden, those difficulties don't appear so overwhelming. We have reason to be thankful for our network of support, medical advancements, and our own incredibly strong willpower. Friend, gratitude makes hope come from sadness.

There is also reframing. We need to shift our perspective, you know? We have the option to use Hepatitis E as a chance for personal development and exploration. It's about overcoming victimisation to demonstrate our resiliency and take charge of our own recovery process. My friend, it's like rewriting the screenplay, and it can truly have an impact.

I now want to offer a few incredible tales of people who have changed their history with Hepatitis E. These tales demonstrate that recovery is achievable regardless of the hand we've been dealt. They serve as evidence that our present situation does not dictate our future. And believe me when I say that these tales will inspire you and inspire you to write your own storey.

But my friend, it's not only about stories. I want you to think deeply and reflect on your life. I have some questions for you that will force you to consider your feelings and convictions. We need to identify any recurring themes or self-limiting ideas that could be preventing us. It all boils down to realising our own narrative and making deliberate decisions that bring about the results we desire.

Oh, and I also received some coping mechanisms and self-care practises designed especially for people with Hepatitis E. We're talking about looking after our mental, physical, and emotional health. It all comes down to treating ourselves with kindness and developing a strong sense of resilience. These methods, which range from mindfulness exercises to connecting with our support system, will enable us to take an active role in our own recovery.

Ultimately, we want to shift our mindset from being helpless victims of Hepatitis E to fierce combatants. We're going to confront those obstacles head-on and recover our agency and purpose. I hope that the techniques and activities I've provided will instil in you a feeling of purpose, resilience, and hope. My friend, it's time to rewrite the storey of our Hepatitis E and make it one of incredible recovery and limitless potential.

So let's get started. Let's own the tale we now tell, reinterpret what happened, and take charge of our own recovery. It's all part of the game: gratitude, changing perspectives, motivational tales, and contemplation. And with optimism, resiliency, and a fire in our bellies, we can rewrite that storey about hepatitis E by emphasising holistic well-being and self-care.

Living Life to the Fullest

I would want to tell you the inspiring tale of Sarah, a young lady who overcome great obstacles with unwavering willpower and tenacity. Imagine a lively, driven soul that is full of dreams and life. Sarah was that. She had recently graduated from college and secured her ideal position at a renowned company. Life was beginning to look good. But then, at the age of 25, everything changed when she was devastatingly diagnosed with hepatitis E.

You can only image her level of shock and dread. Her dreams were crushed, and she was thrown into an unknown world. Sarah experienced a wide range of feelings, including desperation, fury, and a constant wondering of why this had to happen to her. But as time went on, she found herself at a crossroads: she could either focus on the drawbacks of her situation or take use of the chances life still presented.

Sarah started her path of self-improvement and self-discovery with the help of her medical team. In an effort to properly manage her illness, she began investigating various lifestyle changes and self-help methods. Sarah descended into the realm of nutrition and learned how to strengthen her immune system with a balanced diet. She carefully planned her meals and worked with a nutritionist to select foods high in antioxidants, such as fruits and vegetables, lean meats, and healthy fats, to promote the function of her liver. Food turned became the cornerstone of her recovery.

Sarah, however, didn't merely focus on looking after her physical well-being. She realised that complete well-being encompassed her mind, body, and spirit. Sarah explored the world of mindfulness and meditation under the direction of a health and wellness coach. Frequent meditation sessions enabled her to cultivate a profound sense of inner tranquilly and quiet her mind. Her general well-being was greatly enhanced by this newfound tranquilly, which also helped to reduce her stress and anxiety.

Let's be honest now. Sarah's voyage wasn't without difficulties. She experienced disappointments, periods of uncertainty, and days when her symptoms seemed unbearable. But despite everything, she held onto a strong sense of purpose and the conviction that she could control her own fate.

As time passed, Sarah turned her experiences into a positive force and started raising awareness of hepatitis E. She built a supportive network and educated others by sharing her storey and voice. She provided encouragement and hope to people who felt lost and alone through her speaking engagements and participation in support groups.

Sarah is just one of many people who are living well with hepatitis E. Though every storey is different, they are all connected by the resistance to accept a diagnosis. These amazing people overcome hardship and discover meaning and purpose in their path.

It's critical that we never forget that everyone may live life to the fullest, even those who have health obstacles. It's a way of thinking, a decision we make each day to put our health first and take advantage of the opportunities that lie ahead. We can design lives that are joyful, fulfilling, and purposeful if we have the correct support network, make a commitment to self-care, and maintain an optimistic mindset.

As you peruse these motivational accounts of people overcoming Hepatitis E, I urge you to consider your personal experience. What difficulties have you encountered, and how have they influenced you? What goals do you have in mind, and how may you go about pursuing them? Never forget that you are not travelling alone. Seek assistance, establish connections with people who have gone through similar things, and never lose sight of the amazing strength that is inside you.

Let's honour those who have survived with hepatitis E by celebrating their successes. May their experiences serve as a source of inspiration and hope for all of us. Together, let's muster the strength to face life's obstacles head-on with grace and resiliency and seize the chance to live each day to the fullest, no matter what.

Embracing Resilience

Unleashing the Resilient Spirit

It seemed as though everything had turned upside down when I was told I had hepatitis E. I had seen my fair share of sick people in my capacity as a doctor, but receiving a diagnosis was a completely different storey. It was a kick to the gut, and I had to accept that I was now just another sufferer attempting to make my way through this whirlwind of a disease.

It was definitely not a piece of cake, I assure you. Hepatitis E had its hands deep in my gut, and I had to fight daily fatigue, nausea, and this nagging pain in my stomach. I was aware of the technical medical terms, but I was unprepared for the emotional toll this illness would take. I was thrown into the dark of uncertainty all of a sudden, never knowing when or if I would ever get well.

But in the middle of all the confusion, I became aware of one thing: I was still in charge of my own thoughts. I decided to embrace my inner badass and confront this sickness head-on.

I started by flipping the script. I turned my attention from all the things I couldn't accomplish to the things I could. Yes, I had no control over the disease's course or its symptoms, but I did have control over how I responded to it all. I vowed to maintain my optimism and look for the bright spots in every single circumstance.

I also learned about the therapeutic value of self-care. I had taught my patients about it, but until it saved my life, I had never really understood its power. I was very careful to give the things that made me happy and helped me find my zen a higher priority. Those experiences—whether it was going on a leisurely stroll in the park, curving into pretzels during a yoga session, or curling up with a good book—became my pillars, reassuring me that, despite everything, I could still find happiness and serenity.

However, I must say that learning to rely on others was the most important lesson of all. I was always the one giving support because I am a doctor, but during this crazy journey with Hepatitis E, I had to swallow my pride and seek for assistance myself. When I reached out to my family, friends, and fellow doctors, I was blown away by the incredible amount of love and support I received. Even on the worst days, their support gave me the willpower to keep going.

Along this crazy road to recovery, I also dabbled in a variety of complimentary methods. I threw myself into the zen realm of meditation and mindfulness, incorporating those techniques into my everyday routine. Regarding nutrition, I started taking my liver seriously and ate a lot of foods that would cleanse and repair it. I even ventured into the realm of alternative medicine, consulting with hip practitioners who were well-versed in utilising a comprehensive approach to well-being.

Let me be honest with you now: the road to rehabilitation wasn't always easy. Oh doubt, there were hiccups, disappointments, and moments when I really wanted to give up. However, each time I faltered, I would remind myself of the strength of perseverance. Being resilient is about having the willpower to get back up and keep moving forward, not about never falling.

I'm incredibly appreciative of all the lessons this crazy adventure has taught me as I sit here and reflect about it. I've discovered that resilience is a superpower that is innate in each and every one of us. All we have to do is unleash that beast and let it soar.

My advice to you all is to accept your own resiliency and cultivate your inner soul. You are not alone in your fight against Hepatitis E or any other enemy. Seek assistance when needed, schedule self-care activities, and never lose faith in your ability to overcome any obstacle. May you find comfort in your fortitude and may your spirit shine brightly, even in the midst of the fiercest storms, as you set out on your own health path.

Building Resilience Brick by Brick

Resilience is one of those skills that doesn't arise by magic overnight, you know. It's not as though we are endowed with the ability to overcome any obstacle at birth. No, my friend. Resilience is a skill that we develop with practise and experience. You know, it's like building a sturdy brick wall. One brick at a time, each signifying a tactic or instrument that enables us to endure the most trying circumstances and emerge stronger on the other side.

Currently, self-care is one of the most crucial bricks in this resilience wall. Really, give it some thought for a moment. If we disregard our physical, mental, and emotional well-being, how can we possibly expect to be strong and resilient? It's important that we look after ourselves, buddy. It entails eating well, exercising, and giving ourselves time to relax and rejuvenate. Not only that, but we also need to engage in activities that make us happy and relieve stress. Engaging in activities such as meditation, listening to our favourite music, or simply spending time outside are all components of self-care and laying a solid basis for resilience.

But there's still more! Building wholesome relationships is another essential component that we must overlook. I'm telling you, the foundation of resilience is having a support network. When we go through difficult situations, it makes a huge impact. Thus, let us ensure that we foster these significant relationships with the individuals we hold dear. Embrace our support systems of friends, family, and caring communities. Hey, don't overlook the importance of communication. We must be forthright and sincere, ask for assistance when we need it, and extend the same courtesy to others. Creating a network of support is like adding a thick coat of resilience to our wall, my friend!

And you're about to lose your mind over this: adopting a development mentality. Ready for this, are you? It all comes down to having faith that intelligence and skill can be developed via diligence and hard work. Yes, I agree—astounding! it's You see, we strengthen our resilience muscle when we take on new tasks, keep going after we falter, and see failure as a chance for improvement. It's similar to always learning new things and coming up with inventive ways to get past obstacles in life.

Remain focused; we're not quite done yet! We also need to build self-awareness as another brick. It really can change everything to understand our feelings, shortcomings, and talents. It aids in our deft handling of those challenging circumstances. provides us the ability to control our emotions, handle stress, and recognise when it's time to make changes or seek support. It's similar to having an internal compass that points us in the right path and enables us to fall back and get back up stronger.

Alright, buddy, let's speak about coping mechanisms. These serve as our covert weapons against pressure and misfortune. These could be journaling our deepest feelings, practising mindfulness, or just taking deep breaths. Not to mention the things that make us happy and comfortable. We employ these coping mechanisms to enable us to handle difficult situations with poise. Therefore, let's be imaginative, experiment, and expand our resilience toolset.

There's a twist, though! My friend, we must be adaptive and flexible. Being able to roll with the punches and embrace unpredictability is crucial in this constantly changing environment. We cannot be inflexible and set in our ways. Nope, even when things don't go as planned, we still need to be willing to consider new options. It resembles a bamboo tree that bends and sways with the wind as opposed to breaking. I promise you that increased adaptation and flexibility will significantly increase our resilience.

Lastly, but no less important, we must discover our life's meaning and purpose. It functions similarly to fuel to maintain the flame of our resilience. We have a deeper sense of fulfilment and motivation when we work toward goals that are consistent with our values and beliefs and when we have a clear sense of purpose. It is what enables us to persevere, find purpose in the midst of the most difficult circumstances, and emerge from them stronger than before.

Thus, my friend, it's not a simple task to construct resilience brick by brick. It requires work and deliberate practise. But hey, we're developing that resilience foundation like nobody's business by adopting these tactics into our everyday lives. Resilience is constructed one brick at a time, exactly like that brick wall. We're also giving ourselves the fortitude and resiliency to handle whatever that comes our way with every brick.

Coping With Setbacks: Bouncing Back Stronger

I've worked in the medical sector for many years, and I can honestly say that I've seen it all. Patients experiencing really debilitating setbacks in their Hepatitis E journey. I assure you that it is not simple. Anyone would wonder whether there is any hope left after witnessing the abrupt relapses, unforeseen consequences, and mental health toll it takes. The problem is, though, that failures don't spell doom. They are merely obstacles that may be surmounted with the appropriate attitude and techniques.

Reframing unpleasant situations is one of the most effective strategies for dealing with failures. We need to concentrate on the lessons we can take away from this setback rather than obsessing over it. Consider relapses as an example. They have the power to truly depress and exhaust you. However, if we reframe it as an opportunity to reevaluate the treatment plan and make the required changes, it transforms into a step toward improved health.

Allow me to introduce you to Sarah, a patient I will always remember. She was making progress on her Hepatitis E journey, following all the correct procedures. However, she abruptly experienced a flare-up that left her flat. She was, I must say, really frustrated and overwhelmed. We discussed rephrasing the setback in our counselling session. We viewed it as a chance to learn about new treatment choices and obtain further assistance. And you know what? Sarah recovered more powerfully than before. She took back control of her health and her ability to manage her symptoms.

However, that is not our only tactic. Seeing the bright side of things is a highly effective strategy for handling disappointments. There is always something good to hold onto, even in the depth of the most difficult circumstances. Consider James as an example. His deteriorating symptoms forced him to take a leave of absence from work, which was a setback. He was initially devastated. It seemed like everything was against him—his income was gone, his routine was upended. But we discussed such bright spots at our meetings. James came to the realisation that taking time off from work allowed him to spend more time with his family, take care of his health, and take up new, enjoyable activities. He emerged stronger and with a fresh feeling of purpose after adopting a different viewpoint.

And, well, although perspective-shifting and looking for the bright side are beneficial, we also require doable resilience techniques. During failures, self-care is crucial. It is imperative that we tend to our bodies, thoughts, and emotions. This could entail learning how to relax by practising deep breathing, establishing an exercise regimen that works for our circumstances, or even getting in touch with family and support networks. Self-care serves as our shield against the obstacles that setbacks provide. It's what enables us to recover stronger each time.

But what more do you know? We must continue to feel hopeful and optimistic. Although it's normal to feel hopeless and discouraged, we can get past these emotions by maintaining our optimism and self-belief. Set attainable goals, replace those pessimistic thoughts with encouraging ones, and acknowledge and appreciate your little accomplishments along the way. We can keep moving forward and remain dedicated to our rehabilitation if we have optimism in our wallets.

And believe me when I say that having a solid support network is crucial. Reaching out to friends, relatives, or support groups can be quite beneficial when times are difficult. It's like gold to share our difficulties and experiences with like-minded others. They give us validation, comfort, and priceless insights. And who knows, maybe they might offer some useful tips and tactics from their own experiences. They are the ones who can guide us through difficulties so that we can overcome them and emerge even stronger.

In summary, obstacles are a natural part of the Hepatitis E experience, but they do not define us. We can change our perspective, look for the bright side, and put workable resilience tactics into practise. You'll discover all the pointers and information required to transform setbacks into chances for development and resiliency through first-hand accounts and professional guidance. I promise you that obstacles can serve as stepping stones to improved health. We'll prevail if we have the appropriate attitude and tactics.

The Power of Mindset: Shifting Perspectives

You know, it's kind of amazing how our thinking can influence every aspect of our lives. Our attitudes, beliefs, and thoughts all combine to form a mindset that shapes how we respond to the obstacles life presents. Having a growth mentality is like having a secret weapon, I tell you. It all comes down to accepting setbacks as chances for development and education rather than viewing them as failures. It has to do with viewing the glass as half full rather than half empty. The key to navigating life's ups and downs is to take charge of our thoughts and actions.

Let's now discuss hepatitis E. Yes, I realise that this isn't exactly the kind of conversation you have at a dinner party, but stick with me. It turns out that controlling this illness requires having the correct mindset. My friend, it's all about changing our viewpoint. Rather than viewing our diagnosis as a death sentence, we need to view it as an opportunity to develop and change. Really, consider this: our choices about how to react to our situations define us, not the circumstances per se.

How then can we begin to change our perspective? First, though, let's recast the circumstances. We can use our diagnosis as a wake-up call to prioritise our health and make good adjustments, rather than dwelling on all the negative aspects. I promise you that when we adopt that viewpoint, we are completely equipped to take charge of our own path and actively engage in our own recovery.

I had to tell you this storey. It concerns John, a man who was diagnosed with hepatitis E. Man, he was crushed when he first learned. You know, life felt like it hit a brick wall. However, John began making changes with the support of his healthcare team and some mindset coaching. Rather than dwelling on the negative aspects of his health, he chose to concentrate on his mindset, lifestyle, and general well-being.

The things he did will astound you. John began a daily exercise regimen, ate a healthy diet that greatly improved the health of his liver, and even began practising mindfulness to manage his stress. And here's the thing: he made friends with people going through similar things by joining a support group. It was as if he had discovered a tribe who fully comprehended his situation. It had a profound impact.

I have to say, John changed everything with his optimistic outlook. He refused to allow hepatitis E to define him or prevent him from leading a happy life. Nope, he met those obstacles head-on, determined to live each day to the fullest. And what's this? A few researchers looking at how thinking affects chronic illnesses were drawn to his tenacity and will. How about leaving your mark?

Let me now present you with some scientific data to help you decide whether or not the power of mindset has any effect on you. Research from the Stanford University School of Medicine revealed that repeating positive affirmations and maintaining an optimistic outlook really reduced stress and enhanced general well-being. I think that's quite remarkable. Additionally, a different study published in the Journal of Health Psychology revealed that people with long-term conditions who kept a positive mindset were more likely to adhere to their treatment regimens and see improvements in their health. It's true that mindset matters.

So, what are our next steps? Let's get started with some useful activities that can support us in developing the resilient and upbeat mindset necessary to treat hepatitis E with dignity and strength. Initially, we practised gratitude journaling. It's easy; just spend a few minutes every day listing three things for which you are thankful. It assists you in turning your attention from all the bad things in life to the positive things. I promise it will revolutionise the game.

We then heard encouraging affirmations. Make a list of affirmations that you find empowering and repeat them aloud each day. Sayings like, "I can overcome any difficulty because I am strong and capable." You are retraining your brain for resilience and self-belief by repeating these affirmations. It's similar to giving yourself a daily pep talk.

Hey, let's not overlook the importance of visualising. My friend, close your eyes and visualise yourself living a healthy life even after being diagnosed with hepatitis E. Imagine living a happy, fulfilling life, doing everything you enjoy, and feeling well as ever. By utilising the power of your subconscious mind, visualisation creates the conditions for achievement.

Not to mention, we need to look after ourselves. Take part in activities that are good for your health, mind, and soul. It could be as easy as practising mild yoga, meditation, or even engaging in enjoyable hobbies. Setting self-care as a top priority enables us to rejuvenate and strengthen our resilience, which is essential for managing hepatitis E effectively.

Recall that it takes time and practise to change your thinking. It's an adventure, my companion. Thus, treat yourself well and acknowledge each little accomplishment as it comes. You can use your experience with hepatitis E as a chance for personal development, healing, and living life to the fullest if you adopt an optimistic and resilient outlook. Accept the influence of your thoughts and prepare yourself to travel through life with strength and grace.

There you have it: a concise explanation of the power of mindset. It's amazing how our attitudes and thoughts can influence every aspect of our lives. So, my friend, let's harness that optimism. Let us confront hepatitis E head-on with dignity, resolve, and an unwavering spirit. We can change our lives and live each moment to the fullest by utilising the power of our attitude. Go forth and accept it, then. You can do this!

Finding Light in the Darkness: Cultivating Hope

You know, I've seen some incredible things in my years as a medical doctor. And I'm not simply referring to the most recent Grey's Anatomy episode (although that show can be pretty wild). No, what I'm talking about is the impact that a positive outlook can have on a patient's healing process. I promise you, it's like magic.

I've had the honour of personally witnessing the incredible tales of Hepatitis E sufferers who have changed their life. Despite facing significant physical and emotional challenges, these guys haven't let anything stop them. Oh no, they made some delicious lemonade out of those lemons.

Sarah, allow me to tell you about one of my patients. At the age of 25, she was naive to the news that she had contracted Hepatitis E. Could you envision? It completely removed the wind from her sails. The thing about Sarah, though, is that she's a warrior. She embarked on a path of self-discovery and rehabilitation because she would not allow this illness to define her.

But Sarah wasn't working alone. She contacted me and a number of other specialists to assist her devise a strategy. And my goodness, what a gem we came up with. We examined every aspect of her life, including her diet, lifestyle, and emotional well-being. You know, it was a holistic approach. We did not miss a single detail.

And believe me, it was a huge success. In addition to regaining control over her health, Sarah discovered a fresh mission. She began writing a blog on which she told everyone about her experience. Is it really true? She turned into a ray of hope for other Hepatitis E patients. It seems as though her path was about empowering others as much as it was about herself.

I've gained some knowledge in my field of employment. The power of thankfulness is one of those things. It resembles a covert weapon that is not readily apparent. It's amazing how things transform when we give thanks. Those ominous clouds don't look quite so intimidating now. It truly does work like a charm.

Allow me to share with you the power of visualising. It's as if we all possess a superpower that most of us are unaware of. We can literally bring our finest lifestyles to pass by visualising them. I realise it's insane. Still, it's real. This stuff functions.

It's not all sunshine and butterflies, of course. It is not something we can accomplish on our own. We require a safety net. Family, friends, and medical professionals are all very important. However, you know what truly shines? support networks. These people are indispensable. You know, they understand. They are there to cheer you up when you're feeling low since they have experienced the same hardships. It resembles having your very own cheer squad.

Furthermore, remember to look after yourself. It's crucial, particularly if you have a condition like hepatitis E. Exercise, eat healthfully, and attend to your mental well-being. It's important to have strong mental health in addition to good physical health. Believe me, they go hand in hand.

Friends, I've seen it everything. People who have overcome Hepatitis E and changed their lives. It's genuine, not just a pipe dream. And what's this? You are capable as well. By using these techniques, you'll be able to maintain your optimism, foster hope, and find resilience in the face of difficulty.

Hepatitis E can be difficult, yes. However, it's not the end of time. Indeed, this could be the start of something very remarkable. You can find light in the dark and emerge stronger on the other side if you let hope be your guide. So, my friend, keep going. You're only getting started on this adventure, and I can already tell it will be an incredible experience.

Embracing Imperfections: Resilience in Vulnerability

Let's discuss how important it is to accept your flaws and show vulnerability. It's not always simple, but when we succeed, it may truly change our life. Trust me. It's similar to unlocking the ability to withstand adversity, form stronger bonds with others, and have the bravery to take on obstacles like Hepatitis E.

I recall receiving a chronic illness diagnosis once. I had always taken great satisfaction in my physical fitness, so it struck me like a lightning bolt. I was suddenly exposed, with an uncertain and perhaps painful future ahead of me.

I didn't want to be vulnerable at first. I felt ashamed of my illness and believed it to be a sign of weakness. Now, though, what? My sense of loneliness increased when I tried to hide my weakness. Only when I embraced my vulnerabilities and accepted my flaws did I truly connect with people going through similar circumstances.

I've discovered from my own experience that vulnerability is not a sign of weakness. Actually, it's a reflection of how human we all are. We find strength and resilience in our weaknesses because they make it possible for us to access our deepest feelings and establish more meaningful connections with people.

Research confirms this as well. It implies that vulnerability is necessary for resilience in addition to being a positive aspect of being human. Fearless vulnerability researcher Brené Brown says it's about having the guts to be seen and heard, even when we have no control over the result. Being genuine and totally present in our lives, despite uncertainty and perhaps sorrow, is what it means to be vulnerable.

But hold on, how precisely can vulnerability promote resilience? Indeed, we become more receptive to a wide variety of feelings and experiences when we allow ourselves to be vulnerable. This transparency facilitates improved emotional processing, more social support, and the development of coping mechanisms for difficult circumstances.

You know what's even more awesome? Vulnerability strengthens our bonds with other people. Relationships are built on a strong basis when we say to someone, "Hey, I trust you with all my defects and weaknesses." These relationships create a solid support system that can legitimately assist us in overcoming the psychological and physical effects of hepatitis E.

But it's not just that. Accepting our vulnerability also gives us the strength to bravely confront the difficulties posed by hepatitis E. It's similar to reminding oneself, "I will not let this diagnosis to define who I am. I'm stronger than my disease." With this kind of thinking, we can take charge of our well-being, get the help we require, and make choices that are consistent with our objectives and beliefs.

And believe me when I say that I have also witnessed vulnerability work its magic on my patients. Individuals who accept their flaws and allow themselves to be vulnerable exhibit extraordinary fortitude and resiliency. They have a greater propensity to actively participate in their own recovery when they face their diagnoses with courage and truthfulness.

In summary, vulnerability does not equate to weakness. It provides resilience and strength. Accepting our vulnerabilities and flaws invites a wide range of feelings and experiences that can aid in our processing and coping. Also, it strengthens our bonds with one another and provides a solid support system for coping with the difficulties posed by hepatitis E. Most significantly, vulnerability gives us the ability to take charge of our path to wellbeing and health. Therefore, let's welcome our weakness and flaws and allow them to help us become resilient and recover. You can do this.

Redefining Success: Resilience Beyond Achievements

You know, having Hepatitis E really makes you wonder what true success is all about. Success, according to society, is all about attaining goals such as landing the ideal job, obtaining the most expensive degrees, and accumulating a wealth of material belongings. But such definition falls short when dealing with a chronic condition such as hepatitis E. It seems as though we should pause and redefine success. Therefore, I want to explore what resilience actually means in this subchapter and challenge the conventional notion of success. Because, believe me when I say this, success has nothing to do with material possessions; rather, it has everything to do with our inner fortitude, bravery, and resiliency in the face of difficulty.

Let's now discuss the delusion of accomplishments from without. The delusional belief held by society is that external trappings such as fancy titles, high-paying occupations, and social approval are the only factors that determine success. We seem to be inundated with these messages on a daily basis. Now, though, what? A chronic sickness such as Hepatitis E serves as a constant reminder that achievement is much more than that. It's not only about meeting those expectations from without; it's also about how we handle adversity and use it to develop and adapt.

Here's where resilience comes into play. When it comes to living with Hepatitis E, resilience is comparable to the real test of success. It's not about conquering the disease or getting rid of it entirely. Nope. It all comes down to finding the inner fortitude and resolve to roll with the punches. The key to true success is having the willpower to persevere in the face of severe setbacks. It's about overcoming the constraints imposed by the sickness and creating a meaningful life in spite of it.

The truth is, though, that resilience is not a trait we are born with. We can practise this talent over time. Allow me to discuss a few doable tactics that will help you become more resilient to Hepatitis E.

It all starts with accepting positive. Yes, sometimes it's easier said than done. I can assure you, though, that having an optimistic outlook is essential while facing any kind of difficulty, including a chronic illness. Find the good things in life, acknowledge your little accomplishments, and cultivate thankfulness. Changing your point of view has the power to transform.

Next, ask for help. Your ability to connect with and receive support from others will be crucial to developing resilience. Make contact with your loved ones, look for internet communities, and join support groups. Be in the company of understanding individuals who can offer you emotional support and direction. Never undervalue the influence of a solid support system.

Remember the importance of wellbeing and self-care as well. When you have Hepatitis E, it is imperative. Take care of your physical and mental well-being, practise relaxation techniques, and partake in joyful hobbies. Improving your well-being is essential to overcoming this journey and developing resilience.

Adapting to change is another essential component. It's true that Hepatitis E might provide unforeseen challenges. Thus, developing adaptability becomes essential. Accept adaptability, gain experience adjusting to novel circumstances, and hone your problem-solving abilities. Being prepared to roll with the punches is essential when dealing with this illness because life is full of ups and downs.

Now, be sure your goals are reasonable when you set them. Redefining success includes a great deal of that. Establish goals that are in line with your resources and constraints. You'll have a renewed sense of control over your life if you accomplish these goals. It all comes down to discovering fulfilment and success in your own ability.

And believe me when I say that resilience has power. I will provide firsthand accounts in this section of people who have demonstrated incredible fortitude in the face of living with hepatitis E. These tales serve as potent reminders that no sickness can defeat the human spirit. They'll encourage you to choose your own special path to achievement and to have faith in your own resiliency.

As we draw to a close in this chapter, it is evident that success is more than just material accomplishments. The hepatitis E virus forces us to rethink what success is and recognise the real value of resiliency. Thus, let's foster adaptability, prioritise self-care, embrace positivity, get assistance, and establish those doable goals. We'll redefine success on our own terms as we go, comforted by our inner fortitude, bravery, and resiliency. Because that's where real achievement is found—in the unshakeable spirit that keeps us going in the face of difficulties.

The Ripple Effect: Inspiring Resilience in Others

Allow me to take you on a tour. An exploration of the remarkable influence of resilience and its potential to revolutionise the Hepatitis E community. Because of my work as a coach and medical professional, I have personally witnessed it. Being resilient is more than just a term; it's a power that inspires others by sparking their own inner strength and resourcefulness.

Assume the role of a successful executive who receives a surprise diagnosis of Hepatitis E. Fear and doubt pose a threat to your well-being. However, you then come upon a remarkable account of someone who not only made it through Hepatitis E, but flourished in spite of it. You get a ray of optimism from their tenacity, from their capacity to tackle hardship head-on and emerge stronger.

That glint can kindle a fire inside of you, my friend. It forces you to go deep within and discover your own resilience. It encourages you to take charge of your health, look for appropriate medical attention, and modify your lifestyle for the better. As you progress through your personal journey, you also turn into a bright light of hope for those who are going through similar difficulties.

Resilience has an impact on more than just one person's life. Like a network of empowerment, it reaches out to the entire Hepatitis E community. People get together and lift each other up when they share their experiences and coping mechanisms. Every individual possesses a distinct viewpoint and a reservoir of resilience that can be drawn from by others.

However, the effects spread beyond than that. It affects friends, family, and even medical professionals in addition to the Hepatitis E group. Seeing other people's victories and hardships serves as a reminder of our own ability to overcome adversity and endure.

The crucial challenge at hand is how to strengthen the Hepatitis E community's network of support and encourage others to be resilient. I do, however, have some useful advice and techniques up my sleeve, my friend:

Tell us your tale first. Stories have the ability to unite, inspire, and elevate. Thus, show courage and candour about your personal experience with Hepatitis E. Talk openly about the difficulties you've encountered and the methods you've employed to get through them. By disclosing both the victories and the failures, you build a relevant storey from which others can learn.

Be a listening ear next. Sometimes all it takes to encourage resilience in others is a sympathetic ear. Take the time to sit down with someone who is dealing with the difficulties of Hepatitis E and listen to their dreams, disappointments, and worries. Give them your steadfast support and acknowledge their experiences. The ability to recover can vary greatly depending on who you know genuinely cares.

Moreover, provide helpful advice. It takes a community to build resilience. By providing Hepatitis E patients with useful assistance, you enable them to take charge of their health and wellbeing. Assist them in locating suitable medical attention, furnish them with guidance on modifying their lifestyle, or arrange for links to resources and support groups.

Not to mention, resilience-building strategies are important. There are a plethora of research-backed methods and strategies that can improve resilience. Inspire other members of the Hepatitis E community to investigate mindfulness and meditation, partake in physical exercise, cultivate appreciation and good self-talk, and, if necessary, seek treatment or counselling. Giving people these resources gives them the ability to deal with Hepatitis E's obstacles with fortitude and grace.

Finally, cultivate a feeling of belonging. By providing a forum for people to gather, exchange stories, and offer support to one another, the Hepatitis E community may develop a network of resiliency and support. Assemble support groups, engage in online discussion boards, and foster a feeling of community. Recall that there is power in numbers and that people's resilience increases when they get together for a shared goal.

Motivating people to be resilient is a kind and considerate deed. We empower the overall Hepatitis E community by exchanging our stories, offering support, and cultivating a sense of belonging. We empower and uplift others as we empower and uplift ourselves, building a resilient, healthy, and well-being-filled future for everybody. By working together, we can defeat hepatitis E and create a strong future.

A Brighter Future

A Glimpse of Hope

Throughout my career as a physician, I have encountered several courageous individuals who have faced the difficulties posed by Hepatitis E. However, there is one patient in particular whose tale has left a lasting impression on me and serves as a source of inspiration for all others coping with this illness. Allow me to present you to Ravi, a young man in his thirties who was diagnosed with Hepatitis E at a time when his career was booming. Everyone loved Ravi, the software engineer, and his friends and family couldn't get enough of him. Suddenly, everything in his universe was turned upside down.

Imagine this: Ravi is going about his regular life, taking care of himself, and then all of a sudden It's like if someone punched him in the stomach with hepatitis E. You can only image the shock and confusion that followed him, as no one in his family had ever experienced liver problems before. His spirit was broken and he became afraid of what was ahead, as if his entire universe had just collapsed.

Ravi had a difficult battle with hepatitis E. He had to contend with fatigue, excruciating stomachaches, and that terrifying yellowing of the skin. Easy things turned into unachievable missions. Being constantly active, losing control over his body was a difficult pill for him to accept. He was forced to step back from his career and rely more on his family for minor assistance.

However, let me tell you what made Ravi stand out from the crowd: his great energy and never-say-die mindset. He refused to let Hepatitis E to define him, despite the terrible effects it was having on his body and mind. He and his family adhered to all treatment plans, prescriptions, and lifestyle modifications that their healthcare team recommended; they were tenacious in their pursuit of the best medical care. However, what truly ignited Ravi's narrative was his unwavering resolve to investigate supplementary approaches and self-improvement methods that could enhance his healing abilities. He explored a wide range of complementary and alternative therapies, including acupuncture and Ayurveda, to provide his body with the necessary support. And if it didn't make a huge impact, I'll be damned.

With every move he made, Ravi found incredible new opportunities for mindfulness, self-care, and mental health. His tenacity and dedication served as an example for all those around him, including me. As his physician, it gave me great pleasure and optimism to see him advance and make progress. I'll never forget the day he nearly shone with a zest for life that could light up a room when he walked up for his check-up. His blood tests showed a marked improvement, and a full recovery appeared imminent.

Let me tell you, Ravi's tale is unmistakable evidence that hope is a powerful force and that treating Hepatitis E requires more than simply medication. It's about making a complete lifestyle change, taking care of yourself as though it were your work, and getting help psychologically when things go hard. My journey with Ravi showed me that in order to truly and permanently heal, we cannot rely solely on medical solutions. Rather, we must address all potential causes.

And believe me when I say that many people who have experienced the agony of Hepatitis E have been motivated by Ravi's success storey. For those facing their own struggles, his tenacity and resolve provide light in the shadows. We can inspire hope and promise in the hearts and minds of Hepatitis E patients worldwide by sharing tales like Ravi's.

Witnessing Ravi's metamorphosis strengthened my conviction that healthcare should be approached holistically. Taking care of a person's emotional, psychological, and spiritual needs is equally as important as treating their physical ailments. By doing that, we can enable people to take charge of their health and overcome even the most difficult obstacles.

My deepest wish is for Ravi's tale to serve as a ray of hope for everyone lost in the perilous world of Hepatitis E. It serves as a reminder that hope always exists, even in the darkest of circumstances. Thus, let us take a holistic approach to taming this beast, taking care of our health, mind, and soul along the way. Together, let's build a foundation for healing and move forward toward a better tomorrow.

Please keep Ravi's narrative close to your heart as we delve deeper into this book. Allow his path to serve as a reminder to us all of the inner strength we all possess to overcome adversity. Let's work together to find the solution to Hepatitis E as a whole, enabling ourselves and others to face this difficult journey with courage, strength, and an unwavering faith in the power of hope.

Revolutionary Breakthroughs

As a doctor and all, I have to say that staying current on research and treatment choices is essential to comprehending and treating any ailment. And I can assure you that Hepatitis E is not an exception. Understanding this viral infection and developing ground-breaking, hope-filled medicines have brought us a long way.

Determining the various forms of this cunning virus is one of the greatest discoveries in the field of Hepatitis E study. It turns out that we had previously assumed genotype 1 to be the sole cause. That one is seen in impoverished nations with poor access to clean water and sanitation. And here's the thing: new research has completely shocked us by demonstrating that genotypes 3 and 4, which are typically associated with animal viruses, may also infect people. What a turn of events! This finding has improved our knowledge of the virus's mode of transmission and assisted in the development of more effective preventative measures.

But there's still more! Additionally, we've made significant progress in managing hepatitis E. Rest and supportive care were our only options back then because, well, the infection normally went away on its own. Antiviral medication proved to be a game-changer for those suffering from severe symptoms or persistent infections. In clinical trials, two medications—ribavirin and sofosbuvir—have demonstrated some genuine promise. When ribavirin—an all-purpose antiviral medication—was administered to a patient who had both HIV and Hepatitis E, it just so happened that the medication showed promise against Hepatitis E. Another antiviral super hero, sofosbuvir, has demonstrated its efficacy in the treatment of chronic Hepatitis E. For those patients who are suffering the worst of it, there is finally some good news!

Even better, they've developed novel therapeutics that offer us a fresh approach to treating Hepatitis E. For example, are you familiar with monoclonal antibodies? These are these proteins produced in laboratories that, like our immune system, fight off infections. Scientists have developed monoclonal antibodies against the sneaky viral proteins that cause Hepatitis E, which hinders the virus's ability to infect liver cells. How about a thrilling battle! With this medication, a few fortunate patients in early clinical trials have even noticed improvements in their symptoms and a decrease in their viral load. Though further research is necessary to ensure its safety and long-term efficacy, this treatment modifies the way we currently treat hepatitis E.

Furthermore, not simply the treatments have been improved. Also, diagnostic methods have advanced significantly. Prior to today, our methods for identifying viruses or antibodies in blood samples relied on techniques such as polymerase chain reaction (PCR) and next-generation sequencing (NGS). Because PCR can identify even minute levels of viral RNA, we can identify the infection much earlier and begin therapy sooner. Conversely, NGS provides an in-depth analysis of the genetic composition of the virus, enabling us to pinpoint certain mutations and develop more focused therapies. It's like to having a magnifying glass that can disclose every detail about the pathogen. These advances in diagnosis have not only increased precision but also made it possible to tailor treatment regimens to each patient's specific virus profile.

And you know what else? The study of the immune system's reaction to hepatitis e has provided important information for the creation of vaccines. Prevention is always the best option, particularly for high-risk groups. However, creating a vaccination against hepatitis E was not simple. The lack of success with animal models and the unreliability of our lab-grown virus make it difficult to examine. Hey, we managed to crack the code! Currently under development are vaccines that elicit a potent and sustained immunological response. Whereas the other employs an inactivated form of the virus, the first uses a recombinant viral protein. Both have demonstrated some quite encouraging outcomes in clinical trials. Imagine a future in which we can eradicate hepatitis E completely and/or safeguard those at high risk from contracting it. That really is a possibility!

You see, my buddy, the field of Hepatitis E research and therapy has advanced significantly. Our approach to treating this sneaky infection has radically changed as a result of our increased knowledge of the virus's various forms, as well as the creation of novel, extremely powerful medications. Modern diagnostic methods have advanced, and vaccines that have the potential to alter the course of human history are almost here. Though it's an exciting time, we can't take things easy. To provide our patients with the finest care possible, we must be up to date on the most recent research and treatment alternatives. Hepatitis E has a bright future ahead of it, and if we work together, we can pursue a possible treatment.

Unveiling the Hidden

As you may know, I've had the good fortune to have heart-to-heart discussions about living with Hepatitis E with a number of incredible folks. Their stories are eye-opening, I tell you. These courageous people have endured a great deal of discrimination, stigma, and emotional hardships simply to be able to live with this illness.

Sarah was one person who truly touched me. She is a thirty-something woman who was diagnosed with hepatitis E three years ago. It seemed like the entire world had turned upside down when she learned the truth. She was astounded and found it hard to accept. Honestly, who was to blame for her? Managing a chronic condition that is largely taboo is terrifying. Sarah's path has been an emotional roller coaster, filled with hope, sadness, and every emotion in between.

The problem is that Sarah's tale is not special. There are a tonne of folks experiencing similar things throughout the world. Furthermore, what they experience—the discrimination and stigma—is just unfair. You would think that people would be more educated in this day and age, but ignorance and misconceptions are still very common. I mean, this virus doesn't spread through random touch; instead, it spreads through tainted food and drink. Nevertheless, Sarah shared with me tales of how, out of fear, even her own relatives and friends avoided her. It truly is heartbreaking.

Not to mention, the emotional cost is significant. Living with hepatitis e causes you to constantly worry about potential health problems and the future. It's always a concern to consider the potential long-term effects of liver injury. It makes sense why hepatitis E patients frequently experience anxiety and despair. Let me tell you, that's a lot to handle.

The truth is, though, we have the power to change things. We are able to combat discrimination and stigma. The key is education. We can enable individuals to make educated decisions and demonstrate some serious empathy by disseminating factual information about Hepatitis E, including how it spreads and what it actually implies. Don't you think it's about time?

Not to be overlooked is mental wellness. We must fight for these fighters to receive the appropriate support. Resources such as psychosocial therapies, support groups, and counselling can be extremely beneficial for individuals suffering from hepatitis E. Let's equip them with the knowledge and skills necessary to face the emotional obstacles head-on and come out stronger.

In conclusion, we must learn about the realities of having Hepatitis E. The stigma, the discrimination, and the emotional cost must be brought to light. It's time to show compassion, comprehension, and assistance. And the first steps in this process are activism, education, and holistic medical practises. Regardless of the obstacles they encounter, we have the ability to assist these amazing people in leading satisfying lives.

The Ripple Effect

Let me tell you, hepatitis E is no joke. Your liver is affected by this viral infection, which can lead to inflammation and other problems. And where does it prefer to hang out? in areas with poor hygiene and sanitation. Yes, you did hear me correctly. It can be acquired through tainted food or water. Not nice, is it?

However, hepatitis E isn't always fatal. It usually disappears on its own in a matter of weeks or months. But let me tell you, especially for those who are going through it, those weeks or months can seem like an eternity.

The thing that bothers me the most is how it affects relationships. Contemplate it. Family members experience a range of emotions when a loved one is diagnosed with hepatitis E. They feel fearful, anxious, and perplexed. Who is to blame for them? They may retreat or begin to avoid the infected individual since they don't want to get sick. It appears as though they are building a wall out of fear for what might occur. And believe me when I say that wall has the power to strain even the closest of bonds.

I will always remember Sarah, the woman who visited our clinic. Her marriage to her husband was failing, and she had recently received a diagnosis of hepatitis E. The sickness and its implications for their future were too much for him to comprehend. Tension was palpable as miscommunication gave way to complete lack of communication. I was aware that we needed to take action for their overall wellbeing as well as for her physical health.

Furthermore, Hepatitis E can negatively impact both your finances and employment. Imagine yourself working as a chef at a busy restaurant, busting your ass. Then, whoa! You get smacked with hepatitis E like a brick wall. You are unable to work and earn money. It has dual effects. To make matters worse, you start to receive various treatment from people who don't understand the nature of this illness. It seems as though they can catch you with just one glance. Man, it's messed up.

That's how I remember this guy James, he was a chef. He was devastated to learn that he had Hepatitis E. The worry of not knowing how long he would be unemployed was killing him. It was really difficult for him to concentrate on getting healthy. I really did feel sorry for the guy.

The problem with hepatitis E, though, is that it affects entire communities in addition to individuals and those close to them. You can picture the turmoil that exists in areas where this disease is widespread, such as those impoverished nations with little access to healthcare. When an outbreak occurs, the healthcare systems are unable to cope. There is an endless circle of agony, the sickness spreads like wildfire, and people are unable to seek the assistance they require.

In one village I visited, I witnessed it directly. Hepatitis E struck severely because there was no access to clean water or adequate sanitation in the area. Drowning in medical debt, families were finding it difficult to receive the care they required. The village, too? Man, it felt like everything was about to fall apart. It was painful to witness how badly the economy collapsed and how strained social relations became.

Thus, as you can see, Hepatitis E is more than just a medical illness. It tampers with all facets of an individual's existence. To overcome this, we must adopt a thorough strategy. We must address the emotional, social, and financial aspects of health in addition to the medical aspect. The rippling effect must be acknowledged, and action must be taken.

As a medical professional and wellness coach, I'm all about supporting individuals on this journey. Man, I think that a holistic approach is best. We need to empower these Hepatitis E patients and their families—we can no longer only treat the symptoms. We provide nutrition regimens, self-care practises, counselling, and lifestyle modifications. And as we work together, we design a road map for true healing and recovery.

A Ray of Light

Permit me to share with you the amazing effectiveness of support groups for people with Hepatitis E. Believe me, for those battling this illness, these platforms are like a lifeline. They provide a secure environment in where people can meet and discuss their struggles, anxieties, and successes. I assure you, it's a powerful thing.

I recall Sarah, a young lady who, at the age of twenty-five, was diagnosed with hepatitis E. My friend, her journey wasn't an easy one. She was up against mental and physical obstacles that would have knocked anyone flat. Even the easiest chores became difficult for her due to her persistent weakness and exhaustion, and the persistent ache in her abdomen served as a constant reminder of the virus wrecking havoc in her body. She had the impression that she was fighting this battle alone and was losing herself in loneliness.

However, she then discovered this amazing support network created especially for people with Hepatitis E, and let me tell you, it changed everything. She found support from others who understood her issues and didn't pass judgement on her in that group. Their hopes, disappointments, and anxieties were all the same. It turned became her lifeline, a wellspring of support and comprehension. At last, she understood she wasn't fighting this struggle by herself.

Sarah was particularly struck by a storey about a middle-aged man named Alex who, despite all the odds, had recovered from hepatitis E. Despite enduring rigorous therapy and numerous setbacks, Alex emerged from the ordeal stronger than before. In her darkest hours, his storey offered Sarah the comfort and hope she needed. It felt as though there was hope for the future.

Motivated by Alex, Sarah took control of her health and looked into complementary therapies. She jumped into using techniques like acupuncture and meditation and included them in her regimen.

And believe me when I say that there was a huge difference. These holistic methods not only relieved her bodily issues but also gave her the sense of peace and quiet she so desperately needed.

One inspiring example of the resiliency and victory that may be found in the face of Hepatitis E is Sarah's tale. Numerous individuals have overcome the challenges and emerged more resilient than before. These people serve as a reminder that this illness is merely a challenge they have decided to face rather than a reflection of who they are.

And let us not overlook honouring these fighters' individual accomplishments. It's quite simple to concentrate on the restrictions and difficulties associated with Hepatitis E, but we also need to acknowledge the little wins these people experience on a daily basis. While these achievements might not appear significant to others, they mean the world to patients battling Hepatitis E.

Consider John, a man who had run his entire life. He was devastated to learn that he had Hepatitis E. Who is not to be? He could hardly walk, let alone run, from his weakness and exhaustion. Did John, however, let that deter him? No way! To rebuild his strength and endurance, he designed a customised training programme with the assistance of his medical staff. He began by taking short walks and gradually made his way back to jogging. Even if the speed was slower, it was still a victory.

Being able to run again meant far more to John than just improving his physical condition. It was evidence of his steadfast attitude and resolve. He refused to let Hepatitis E determine how he lived his life, in spite of all the obstacles and disappointments. His experience serves as a reminder to all of us that, in the face of difficulty, we are all capable of finding the inner strength to persevere.

In the worst of circumstances, these tales of resiliency and victory serve as a beacon of hope. They tell us that, despite the appearance of gloom, there is always hope that is just waiting to be found. It could be discovered in a consoling and empathetic support group, or it could be discovered in individual accomplishments that surpass the constraints imposed by the illness.

As a physician and wellness coach who works regularly with Hepatitis E patients, I have the amazing honour of seeing these instances of resiliency and victory firsthand. I've witnessed people overcome seemingly impossible challenges and come out stronger than before. And trust me when I say that it's these tales that motivate me to carry on with my work of offering advice and assistance to people suffering from hepatitis E.

I will go into the methods and approaches that people might use to find their own beacon of hope in the pages that follow. We'll discuss diet and nutrition, self-care practises, therapy, psychology, and adjustments in lifestyle. It will serve as a thorough management guide for hepatitis E. However, I want to take a minute to recognise and celebrate the victories and acts of resilience that give us hope and inspire us to keep fighting before we go into all the technical details.

So, my dear readers, may these tales serve as a reminder that you are not alone if you have Hepatitis E. The prospect of a better future never goes away. Allow these tales to serve as a roadmap for your arduous path to recovery and well-being.

The Road Ahead

Hi everyone! Imagine that I am a medical doctor who also coaches people in health and wellbeing. I am committed to providing my patients with the most up-to-date information and treatments accessible. And believe me when I say that the field of hepatitis E is one that is constantly changing. Scientists and researchers are working around the clock to comprehend this illness, develop fresh therapies, and discover an actual cure!

The creation of a Hepatitis E vaccination is one field that is receiving a lot of interest. There isn't an approved vaccine that is generally accessible just yet. Don't worry, though; a number of prospective vaccinations are undergoing clinical studies. These bad guys are meant to kick the ass of Hepatitis E, either by preventing infection or at least lessening the severity of the symptoms. Everyone is eagerly awaiting the trial findings because, should a vaccine be developed, the global burden of Hepatitis E would be greatly reduced.

But wait, there's still more! Researchers are looking into novel antiviral medications in addition to vaccines to treat Hepatitis E. The ones we now have occasionally collapse, particularly in extreme circumstances. Therefore, researchers are developing medications that precisely target the virus's weak points to prevent it from proliferating and spreading throughout the body. Let me explain this fancy scientific jargon for you: these tailored medications are demonstrating promise in the lab and in preliminary trials. We might soon have some further weaponry against Hepatitis E with further study and testing.

And let's not overlook diagnostics, please! Researchers are looking for quicker and more accurate methods to identify hepatitis E. Quick diagnostics that can quickly identify this cunning virus are being developed. Furthermore, they are developing portable medical equipment that can be utilised in areas where access to high-quality healthcare is limited. It is imperative that individuals receive prompt diagnosis, regardless of their location!

But here's the problem, buddy: let's discuss the long-term implications. The majority of Hepatitis E patients resolve on their own with little difficulty. Phew! However, there's a developing theory that certain people may develop chronic Hepatitis E. And that's unfortunate. It may result in cirrhosis, liver fibrosis, and in the most terrible of situations, liver cancer. Therefore, we need to understand this chronic condition and come up with strategies for managing it. Without a doubt, it will change the game for the patients.

Oh, and when it comes to Hepatitis E, those with compromised immune systems and expectant mothers should pay particular care. They may require extra-special attention and care because they are somewhat more susceptible to the illness. To determine what puts these populations at danger and how we can significantly improve their quality of life, research is moving forward at a rapid pace.

Ultimately, as new information regarding Hepatitis E emerges, it is critical that patients become informed and involved in their own care. Patients can accelerate their healing process and make well-informed decisions about their therapies by keeping up with the most recent research and developments. As healthcare professionals, we also need to stay current and provide patients with evidence-based care. Cooperation, my friend! We cannot defeat Hepatitis E unless researchers, medical professionals, and patients band together. Imagine a time in the future when the effects of this illness are mitigated, or better yet, eradicated entirely!

Ultimately, there are a lot of opportunities and potential advancements on the path to monitoring and curing hepatitis E. More study into vaccinations, antiviral medications, diagnostics, and long-term impacts will improve patient outcomes and quality of life.

Thus, let's educate ourselves, become involved, and move forward in the direction of a safer and more promising future. I really hope you're in on this as well!